AF352230

WOMEN GAIN A PLACE IN MEDICINE

THE HISTORY OF SCIENCE

Prepared under the general
editorship of Daniel A. Greenberg

WOMEN GAIN A PLACE IN MEDICINE

by Edythe Lutzker

McGRAW-HILL BOOK COMPANY

NEW YORK • TORONTO • LONDON • SYDNEY

For the young people of this generation and those to follow

PICTURE CREDITS

WOMEN GAIN A PLACE IN MEDICINE

ISBN 07–039115–7

Library of Congress Catalog Card Number: 69–17185

234567890 VBVB 754321

CONTENTS

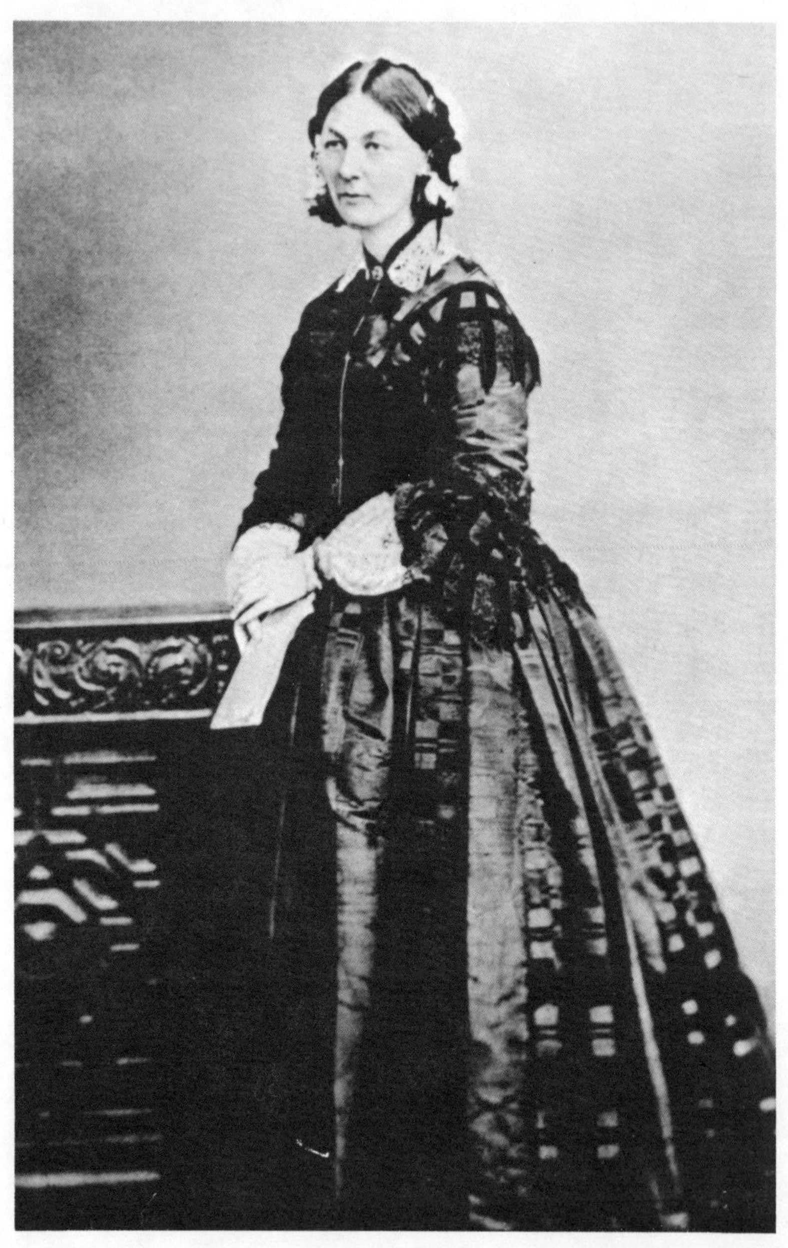

Florence Nightingale (1820–1910)

This book has five heroines; in telling the story of how this handful of courageous young women sought, in the second half of the nineteenth century, to enter the medical profession—and paved the way for countless others—I have tried to help young readers appreciate the difficulties they encountered on their rugged, uphill path. They were confronted with many obstacles, many opponents, and to make these more understandable, I have tried, for example, to clarify the complicated structure of the University of Edinburgh, where this brave band of women tried so hard to get a medical education. I have also sought to give readers a look at the general condition of medical education in America, continental Europe, and Great Britain at the time of these daring pioneers and to introduce them to our heroines' well-known (and sometimes *un*known) forerunners—the mysterious James Barry, the great Elizabeth Blackwell, among others.

Our bold young women were no doubt discouraged at times by the setbacks they so often met with in their fight to become doctors. But did they abandon the battlefield? Not they. Did they, by their determination and perseverance, help to change the pattern of thinking about the place of women in society, in higher education in universities, in medicine, even in the home? It would not be an exaggeration to say that they did.

I hope by my efforts to have provided young people with vibrant examples of dedication, from which uncounted generations to follow have been, and will continue to be, the beneficiaries.

Does that mean that all traces of discrimination or prejudice against women in medicine no longer exist? Of course they still exist. But there is no doubt that these have gradually diminished in intensity to a large extent. The roadblock now is the promotion of women to policy-making positions. It is a good fight!

Women make up more than half the population of the world; they represent a huge reserve of potential talent that can and should be placed in the service of humankind. This generation can set the example for those to come by taking up this challenge and pointing the way to a better, more useful and rewarding life, that will not be measured only by the acquisition of more gadgets, but by the expansion of women's role within the family as well as of cultural, economic, political, and social horizons within society as a whole.

E. L.

An obstetrics textbook published in Philadelphia in 1848 contained the following information about women: "The great administrative faculties are not found in women. . . . [Woman] reigns in the heart. . . . Home is her place, except when, like the star of day, she deigns to issue forth to the world, to exhibit her beauty and her grace . . . and then, she goes back to her home, as the sun sinks in the west, and the memory of her presence is like a bright departed day. . . ." And then the author concluded: "She has a head almost too small for intellect but just big enough for love."

Somewhat less flattering in his appraisal of women was a British physician—a certain Dr. Bennet—who had this to say about women doctors in 1870 in a letter published in *The Lancet*, the leading British medical journal: ". . . as a body they are sexually, constitutionally, and mentally unfitted for the hard and incessant toil, and for the heavy responsibilities of general medical and surgical practice." He went on to recommend that the women might be admitted to the practice of midwifery, but "in a subordinate position as a rule," and then he set forth his general conclusions: "The principal feature which appears to me to characterise the Caucasian race, to raise it immeasurably above all other races, is the power that many of its *male* members have of advanc-

1.

"But to None Others"

ing the horizon of science, of penetrating beyond the existing limits of knowledge—in a word, the power of scientific discovery. I am not aware that the female members of our race participate in this power, in this supreme development of the human mind; at least I know of no great discovery changing the surface of science that owes its existence to a woman of our or of any race. What right then have women to claim mental *equality* with men?"

If this was the view of some men in the nineteenth century of women and their capabilities, it was certainly not the view held by certain women. This century was to see—in America, in Great Britain—a great battle as women, in the face of opponents who held opinions such as these, sought to enter the profession of medicine.

The Hippocratic oath, which is still administered to both men and women today (and incidentally probably wasn't written by Hippocrates at all but by someone else several hundred years after Hippocrates' death) had spoken of a pious brotherhood of physicians, and in unmistakably masculine terms had included these words: "I will impart a knowledge of the art [of medicine] to my own sons and those of my teachers and to disciples . . . but to none others." If some of the sanctity of the profession had disappeared over the years, still the idea of a male proprietorship remained. In fact, for most of the nineteenth century, women, especially in Britain and America, were excluded from medicine by every possible means, whether explicit or implicit, that could be contrived by medical colleges and universities, by the medical profession, and even by governments themselves. Medical journals refused to publish articles written by women. (Some women submitted articles but used their initials only. Some used assumed male names.) Medical societies and groups barred women from membership and from access to their libraries.

In short, medicine (with the exception, as we shall see, of

midwifery) was something of a male preserve, and for years no one had challenged this idea. But then, in the nineteenth century, times began to change, and a few eager—and determined—young women appeared on the scene.

Some wanted to bring comfort to the sick, but lacked the knowledge that would enable them to do so. Some could not resign themselves to a life of homemaking and child rearing only, and indeed were convinced that medical knowledge would, whenever they married and had children of their own, be a great help in caring for their families. Some had a missionary zeal; they wanted to go to far-off countries where life was quite primitive and where diseases that had already been brought under control in their own countries were still stalking at will and taking a great toll, especially among the women and children. Rarely did women plan to minister to others than women and children, even in some of the European countries. And it may even be said that some were motivated to study medicine to convince men, both young and old, that anything they could do women could do as well—and sometimes even better.

It was not very difficult for young women to become nurses. Florence Nightingale's service during the Crimean War in 1854 had stirred up public feeling about the shocking loss of life as a result of the complete lack of nursing or the very poor nursing of the wounded and the outrageous lack of drugs, hospital equipment, and even the most elementary attempts at cleanliness. Training for nurses really began just about then, and its scope was quite limited. But as time went on, nurses were required to take special courses in all sorts of subjects that, with developments in medical science, were considered to be indispensable.

Having overcome the initial resistance she experienced when she undertook her crusading work in the Crimea, and having demonstrated the validity of her methods during the war, Florence Nightingale convinced the British authorities that more attention must be paid to the recruiting, training, and building of a corps of nurses for duty at home and in the far-flung British Empire. Her struggle was certainly not an easy one, but she won her fight. A nursing school soon became a part of every or almost every hospital in Great Britain. And where none existed, it was on the agenda for the foreseeable future. Doctors raised no objections to nurses carrying on their duties in all wards of the hospitals, whether the beds were occupied by men or by women. Nor did they object to the nurses' long hours, hard work, and low pay.

Their entire attitude changed, however, when women showed an interest in becoming qualified physicians—and in university educations that would give them the required scientific knowledge. But before we turn to the first woman doctors, let us take a brief look at the role women had played in medicine throughout history.

From biblical times women have tended the sick, inside their homes and outside, when they were called in by neighbors to help or even to undertake by themselves the deliveries of new babies into the world. The only knowledge they had at their command, in most cases, was the experience acquired over the years. They were the midwives of the poor and rich alike, of peasant women and of queens. They had no theoretical training in any of the relevant branches of medicine, for the reason that none existed. In fact, the stereotype of the midwife in the seventeenth, eighteenth, and nineteenth centuries was a combination of advanced age, ignorance, drunkenness, and filth—in short, an old, toothless hag, a necessary evil. Like all stereotypes, it was an unjust, untrue composite of some of the worst characteristics of the minority of midwives.

During the Cromwellian wars in England, i.e., in the middle of the seventeenth century, there was a concerted attempt among midwives to acquire some training that would help them in what often turned out to be a struggle between life and death—sometimes of the mother, sometimes of the child, sometimes of both. The deaths of women in childbirth and of children at birth reached astronomical figures. The medical education of doctors did not include obstetrics until the late 1890s because people believed that since childbirth was a natural process, nature would take its course no matter what. In addition, it was the prevailing religious attitude that if mother and child lived, God be praised! If either mother or child died, God's will be done! Depending on nature and divine will in this way made unnecessary a study of the physiological process of childbirth. Of course, in normal cases, problems did not arise. But how was an untrained midwife to know just when a case became abnormal? And what was she to do at the moment she observed something that was not familiar to her from previous experience? She might call a doctor, if one was available and willing to come, and his knowledge of anatomy might be useful in recognizing an unusual condition, and then he might do what he thought that particular situation called for. But he usually depended on the method of trial and error. If he was lucky, he might save the mother, even though she might be left with internal abnormalities that would give her trouble for many years to come. The child, if it survived, might be scarred for life or might even be crippled owing to brain damage at birth. In any case, doctors' interference was known as "meddlesome midwifery," and it was frowned upon in the profession, even when successful.

In 1827, the president of the Royal College of Physicians in London wrote that midwifery was "an act foreign to the habits of a gentleman of enlarged academic education." That he was not alone in that point of view even seven years later is demonstrated by the statement of an eminent surgeon to a parliamentary committee that "it is an imposture to pretend that a medical man is required at a labour." These are not casual remarks by uneducated people. There is strong feeling expressed in both statements. The astonishing thing is that such statements were made despite the fact that the wives of doctors were not immune to the hazards of childbirth. One wonders how and why the medical profession was content to let matters rest in that state of affairs for so long. And when they finally did anything about it, it was only as the result of a great public outcry against the quackery and incompetence of doctors and a demand for changes in university curricula and the training of medical faculties—in short, for medical reform to correct dishonesty, ignorance, and malpractice among practitioners and inside the teaching institutions and examining bodies.

Let us go back to the midwives, because it took a long time for the majority of women to turn to male doctors. In their favor, let it be said that the most conscientious among the midwives did not overlook their need for greater knowledge, and tried in many ways to acquire it. For example, the earliest attempts to teach midwifery in England occurred in the first quarter of the seventeenth century. A family of physicians had invented the forceps, which reduced the danger of infant and maternal mortality, but they kept this instrument and its use a family secret for many generations. However, they offered to instruct midwives in the use of it without divulging the secret of its construction. They were accused of trying to establish a monopoly, and nothing came of their efforts.

Oddly enough, the University of Edinburgh, which, as we shall see, was to be the scene of some of the fiercest battles over the right of women to study medicine, created the first chair of midwifery in 1726, but medical students were not obliged to study that subject. In fact, the principal of the University stated that "it was hardly contemplated in those days that medical students should go through a course of obstetrics, the whole practice and profession of which was then left to females." There could be no more convincing evidence that not only were the midwives denied training, but the male medical practitioners were uninformed, ill-informed, and, what is worst of all, uninterested!

How did the situation in Great Britain differ from that in other countries? As late as 1872, England was the only European country that did not supervise the practice of midwifery. In every other country, midwives were instructed by the state, then licensed and supervised. Florence Nightingale wrote in 1881 that "it is a farce and mockery to call [women practicing midwifery] midwives or even . . . nurses. . . . France, Germany, and even Russia would consider it woman slaughter to 'practice' as we do."

When the Midwives Institute was finally established in London in 1881 "to raise the status of midwives and petition Parliament for their recognition," the bill it drafted and supported failed to pass. A statement in 1889 by the recently created Medical Council acknowledged that "the absence of public provision for the education and supervision of midwives is productive of a large amount of grave suffering among the poorer classes," and it pressed for Government passage of a measure providing "for the education and registration of midwives."

There can be little doubt that young girls were aware of the dangers their mothers faced with each pregnancy. Indeed, many were left motherless quite early in their lives. Many witnessed the awful goings-on in the house during the hours when the life-and-death battles were being fought, since most often women had their children at home and not in hospitals (though being in a hospital was itself not an unmixed blessing). And what about the fears that must have seized the young girls as they thought of the future, when they themselves might be undergoing the ordeal of childbirth?

Should we then be surprised that some of them desired to study medicine, to serve women and children? Perhaps some even wished to bring to the attention of medical faculties and doctors the fact that they were guilty of ignoring the well-being of even their own wives and sisters by neglecting to dig deeply into the reasons why so many women died during a natural physiological process. This great gap in medical knowledge and practice was a challenge that evoked a vibrant echo in the hearts and minds of some young women.

For some, the concern for tending to women involved more than childbirth alone. With Victorian prudishness and misplaced modesty, women often failed to seek medical help at all if it meant disclosing certain "delicate matters" to male doctors. Women physicians were needed to encourage women to become patients while they could still be healed.

Perhaps somewhat different reasons lay behind the decision of a certain very young girl to study medicine, but in any case it is a matter of recorded history that in 1812 a girl who had assumed the disguise of a man was awarded a medical degree from the University of Edinburgh—when she was fifteen years old! Her name was Dr. James Barry. She was the first woman doctor in the British Isles. She cut her hair and wore trousers all her life. She joined the British army in 1813 as a hospital assistant and was promoted to assistant surgeon as a reward for distinguished service during the Battle of Waterloo. She kept the secret of her sex throughout her life. Even her male servant, who accompanied her to many parts of the British Empire, including South Africa, Canada, and the West Indies, did not know that she was a woman. In South Africa she was staff surgeon and medical adviser to Lord Charles Somerset, Governor of Cape Town. She was quarrelsome and was frequently arrested for breaches of discipline. But the Governor, who considered her a very skillful physician, usually overlooked her behavior and did not punish her very severely. Seven years before her death her name appears in official army lists followed by her title, Head of Inspectors-General of Hospitals. That was the highest position in the service.

She left instructions that no autopsy was to be performed

when she died. But the medical authorities paid no attention to those instructions when her death was reported in July, 1865, and they discovered that she had played the part of a man for over fifty years. Her death certificate was marked "male" and so was the inscription on her tombstone. The British officials were not going to admit that such a deception had been carried out—and that they had known nothing about it! The word "male" on her death certificate and on her tombstone officially confirms the impersonation. (Although the true story finally did leak out, we do not know to this day the real name of this mysterious lady surgeon.)

While Dr. James Barry was serving in the British army, another woman was attempting to make her mark in medicine, but in her own right, as a woman—although she may have used a trick or two, as we shall see. This woman was Elizabeth Blackwell, of America.

She was born in England in 1821 and was one of eight children. Her father, Samuel, had business reverses in England so the family decided to emigrate to America, which they did in 1832. He was, fortunately, a strong believer in educational opportunities for his daughters as well as for his sons. We know that Elizabeth decided rather early in her life that she wanted to study medicine. She took every opportunity to improve her knowledge, reading everything she could put her hands on. With money she earned at other jobs, she engaged private tutors, and when she felt that her preliminary education would be sufficient for admission to a medical school, she began to send applications to colleges and universities for admission. She got little encouragement and was, in fact, rejected. Then, one day, a medical school in Geneva, New York, agreed to admit her. Here is where the trick comes in, for some say that her application was signed with her initial only, E. Blackwell, so it was not known that she was a woman until she appeared at Geneva Medical College to begin her studies.

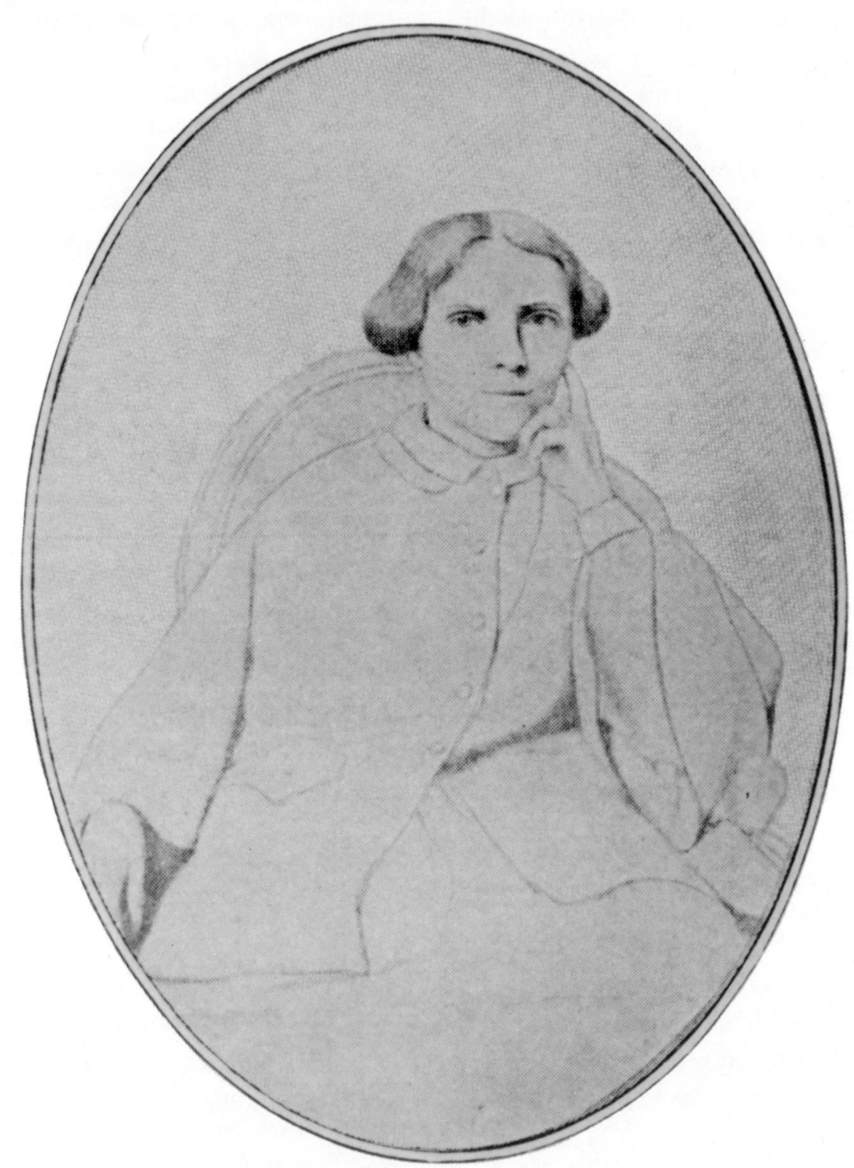

Elizabeth Blackwell (1821–1910)

The matter of Elizabeth's admission was placed in the students' hands oddly enough (perhaps because the college faculty didn't want the responsibility of rejecting her and hoped the students would do it for them). In an idealistic resolution the all-male student body declared that "to every branch of scientific education the door should be opened equally to all," and so they had extended to her their "unanimous invitation," making Geneva the only medical college in the country that could boast a woman student.

It was not an easy moment for Elizabeth when she first faced the student body. Years later, a doctor who had been a student at the time described the scene as the dean led her to the platform and introduced her to the assembled student body: "The class, numbering about 150 students, was composed largely of young men from the neighboring towns. Usually they were rude, boisterous, and riotous beyond comparison. On several occasions the residents of the neighborhood sent written protests to the Faculty threatening to have the college indicted as a nuisance if the disturbances did not cease. During lectures it was almost impossible to hear the professors owing to the confusion."

When Elizabeth appeared on the platform to be introduced to her "hosts," no doubt they were quite surprised to see, not the Amazon they had expected, but quite a small young lady. She was dressed very simply and appeared to be quite shy, but her face bore an expression of determination. "Her entry into the Bedlam of confusion acted like magic on every student," recounted her onetime classmate. "Each hurriedly sought his seat, and the utmost silence prevailed. For the first time a lecture was given without the slightest interruption, and every word could be heard as distinctly as it would be if there had been but a single person in the room. The sudden transformation of this class from a band of lawless desperadoes to gentlemen by the mere presence of a lady proved to be permanent in its effects."

Elizabeth's gentle manner, and the quiet way she went about her work, soon became known in the town. The school came in for quite a bit of publicity, which was not entirely unwelcome, in connection with its admission of the first woman medical student.

At final examination time the records showed that Elizabeth was the best in the class! And yet the officials of the college hesitated about granting her a medical degree! It was unprecedented. Elizabeth had earned, however, the unqualified support of the professors, and they insisted that, having done everything required for the degree and, moreover, having passed every course with honors, she was entitled to the degree. On January 23, 1849, crowds of people came for the graduation ceremony, and they were full of smiles, especially the women. Elizabeth did not want to be the center of attention, so she chose to sit with her brother, who had come up for the event, instead of walking in with the procession. When all the students had walked up to receive their diplomas, Elizabeth was called up alone, the last one. She walked up to the platform with great dignity, stood before the college president, and bowed slightly as she prepared to receive her diploma. And the president of the college, handing the rolled-up parchment to her, took off his mortarboard to Dr. Elizabeth Blackwell.

Elizabeth turned to go and then, suddenly, turned back to face the president. "Sir, I thank you," she said. "By the help of the Most High, it should be the effort of my life to shed honor upon your diploma!"

And this she did. Since, as a woman doctor, she could not receive hospital training in America, she decided to go to Paris, where she won honors in postgraduate work. In 1857 she founded the first school of nursing in America; in 1866 she opened the New York Infirmary in one of the crowded neighborhoods on the lower East Side of Manhattan where the poorest immigrant population lived. In 1871 she started an organization in England called the National Health Society for the teaching of health habits, hygiene, and disease prevention.

Elizabeth Blackwell died in 1910. By then she had also organized a women's association for nursing and relief during America's Civil War, and had made a major contribution, which we shall speak more of later, in England to the cause of women in medicine.

In America, at mid-century, the women's rights movement, and along with it the cause of women in medicine, had been gathering momentum. In 1850 the Woman's Medical College of Pennsylvania was founded in Philadelphia. In 1848 a Boston medical doctor had established there a school for training midwives, which did not, however, satisfy those women who wanted a more complete education in medicine. Some women formed "Ladies' Physiological Reform" societies and heard lectures on anatomy and physiology given by women who had received some medical training. A few of the women who enrolled in medical college at that time did so with the idea of giving lectures in sex education and general hygiene. Large groups of young working girls and women were reaching out for more knowledge, wherever and however it became available, and they took advantage of these scattered attempts by women lecturers to fill in the wide gaps in their knowledge about sanitation, personal hygiene, care of children in the home, etc. The road that led to medical degrees for women in America in the second half of the nineteenth century was not to be an easy one, but at least the first steps in America had been taken.

In continental Europe, things were somewhat better. By the second half of the nineteenth century, most countries, as we have mentioned, had set up schools for midwives, supervised by the governments and some medical men.

The universities of Bologna and Salerno in Italy, to mention just two, admitted women for medical studies (they had been admitted as early as the fourteenth century), and some women were even on their teaching staffs as professors. The hospitals gave them the clinical experience they needed to become competent doctors.

In Paris, France; Zurich and Bern, Switzerland, the same situation existed in the universities for medical studies and degrees, and in clinical work.

In Russia, most backward of modern countries until almost the middle of the twentieth century, we find the name of a woman who, in 1869, had already graduated from a medical college and held a medical degree. Now it is true that her university career was not completed with the sanction of the czarist government. In fact, she was smuggled into the various classes with the help of students and professors who realized her extraordinary talents and great desire for learning. But when she was given her degree at graduation time, her record was so outstanding that not only was she given a high academic honor, but her fellow students carried her around on their shoulders as a tribute to her success in overcoming the serious obstacles she had met all along the way. Soon after, however, the Government issued a decree prohibiting other women from gaining admission to universities. That restriction was lifted in the 1870s. The first medical school for women was opened in St. Petersburg in 1872; it was one of six medical academies in existence in that city. From 1878 to 1888 nearly seven hundred women earned medical degrees there.

When Elizabeth Blackwell became America's first woman doctor, the British magazine *Punch* printed these verses:

> Young ladies all of every clime
> Especially of Britain
> Who wholly occupy your time
> In novels or in knitting,
> Whose highest skill is but to play
> Sing, dance, or French to clack well,
> Reflect on the example, pray,
> Of excellent Miss Blackwell.

The poem went on to extoll the virtues of having a "sister, wife, or daughter" as family physician. But *Punch* is a magazine of satire and humor, and the poem did not really reflect what the rest of England was thinking. Perhaps it was almost a cruel joke, for when those "sisters, wives, and daughters" sought to enter medicine, they met the most hardened opponents and the harshest treatment from the universities and many medical men. Of all the countries where women were trying to enter medicine at that time, perhaps the greatest challenges—and therefore, perhaps, too, the greatest victories—are to be found in Great Britain and in the stories of the women who blazed the trail into the medical profession there.

Sophia Jex-Blake was the first; she was joined by Edith Pechey, Mrs. Isabel Thorne, Matilda Chaplin, and Mrs. Helen Evans—and soon by others. These young women accepted the challenge offered by British medical men and universities with determination, despite the great cost in endurance as well as in money! Moreover, to their everlasting glory, they acquitted themselves with honor, dignity, and exemplary performance. Most important, they won many men and women, inside and outside the profession, over to their side in the long, uphill, soul-searing battle from which they emerged victorious after more than a decade.

But before we turn to their own stories, let us look first at the England of their time.

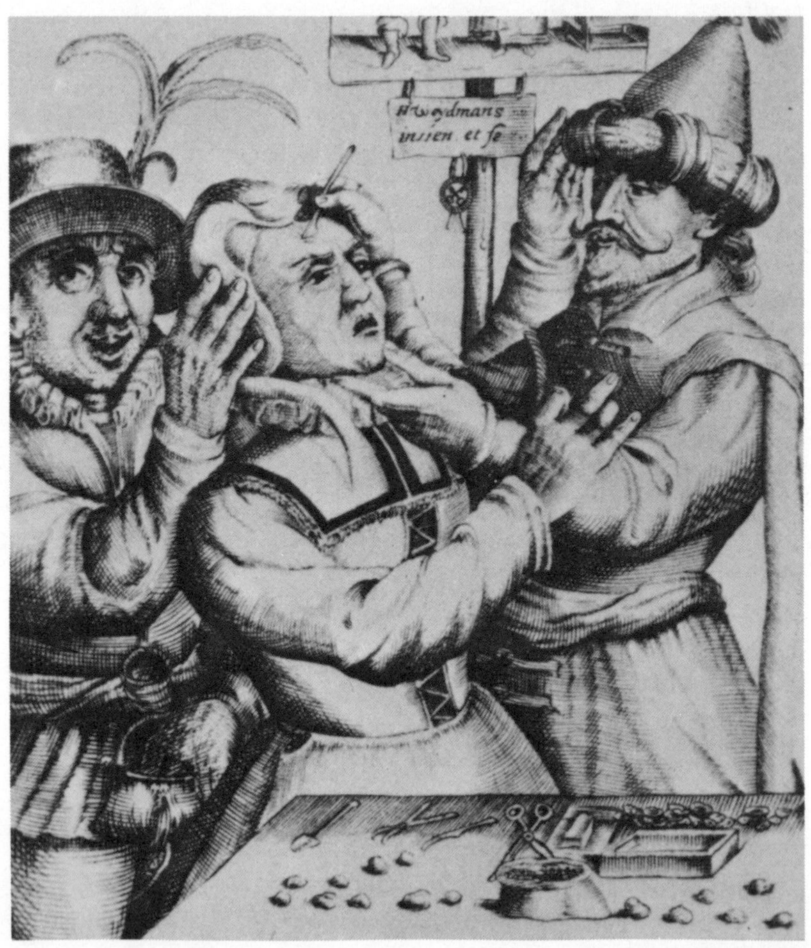

All sorts of quacks promised complete cures for every imaginable malady, and prior to the nineteenth century the insane were treated brutally, as demonstrated in this old print entitled Operation for Stones in the Head *by H. Weydmans.*

What kind of life could a woman expect in nineteenth-century England? This century was, as we shall see, a century of internal ferment for England, and it was an age of reforms, but reforms that often came only long after the need for them had become desperate. If the status of women was not to receive much improvement from these reforms, at least industry and also the medical profession were to see some long-needed changes finally made.

First, though, let us look at the political situation. For most of the nineteenth century, it was—ironically, perhaps—a woman who ruled England: Queen Victoria, who enjoyed an unusually long reign, from 1837 to 1901.

Victoria was born at Kensington Palace on May 24, 1819. She was the only child of Princess Victoria Mary Louisa of Saxe-Coburg-Gotha and Edward, Duke of Kent. A month later, on June 24, 1819, she was christened, after some disagreement about what to name her. Czar Alexander I, who was to be godfather, pressed his choice of Alexandrina, and so she was named. (Had it not been for her father's request that she be given another name as well—and the Czar's quick allowance that she might be called after her mother, Victoria, but this as a *second* name only— the period of her reign might well be known today as the "Alexandrinian" era.)

2.

All This for A Woman!

Six weeks later the princess was vaccinated. This was the first vaccination ever performed on a member of the royal family.

Victoria's education was supervised by her favorite uncle, Prince Leopold, and it was his judgment that if she knew, in early childhood, that she would be queen, she might become vain, proud, and unmanageable. And so not until she was twelve years old was she told that she would wear the Crown of Britain.

On the morning of June 20, 1837, at 5 A.M., the Archbishop of Canterbury and a nobleman brought word to Kensington of the king's death.

Later that morning the Privy Council assembled to swear allegiance to the new queen, seated on the throne. As two of her elderly uncles approached the throne and were about to kneel, according to the custom, Victoria blushed, rose, came down the stairs, and kissed them both without allowing them to kneel.

On June 28, 1838, the coronation took place. It was, by all accounts, the most touching ceremony ever performed in Westminster Abbey. Earlier, England had been ruled by four queens, all middle-aged and ungainly and all objectionable on religious or other grounds to some sections of the population. The young Queen Victoria, however, had no enemies, except, perhaps, a few Chartist reformers. The country was at peace. It was prospering when her reign began. As it moved from the Palace through London's streets to Westminster Abbey, the royal procession made the finest show that had ever been seen. To view these ceremonies 400,000 visitors came from England alone. Three foreign ambassadors were present, and the one from Turkey was especially bewildered; he kept muttering under his breath, "All this for a woman!"

A year before Victoria became queen, her uncle, who had meanwhile become King Leopold I of Belgium, had visited Kensington Palace with his two sons, the princes Albert and Ernest. He favored a marriage between Victoria and Albert, who had been born in the same year as Victoria, and who was also her first cousin. There were some who expressed disapproval of the match, but Victoria paid no attention to them because, as she wrote at one point to her uncle, "Albert's beauty is most striking, and he is so amiable and unaffected—in short, very fascinating. I love him more than I can say."

Public announcement of their engagement was received with great enthusiasm and joy. They were both twenty years old and in love!

On the tenth of February, 1840, Queen Victoria and Prince Albert were married in the Chapel Royal, St. James's. For the twenty-one years of their married life they were a fine example of the ideal married couple. By 1857, their family had grown to nine children—four sons and five daughters. Less than a year later the Princess Royal was married, and the others followed at various intervals up to 1885.

Prince Albert was particularly interested in natural science, philosophy, and economics, as well as music, art, and gymnastics, especially fencing, and he was of great help to Queen Victoria in the management of Britain's domestic affairs. He favored many of the reforms so badly needed in England at that time and initiated several others. The Queen placed great confidence in him and relied on his advice. In affairs of state his prudence contributed much toward raising the tone of the court and the influence of the Crown.

Albert was elected president of the British Association for the Advancement of Science, delivering his inaugural address in 1859. His early death in December of 1861, at the age of forty-two, was a terrible blow to the Queen. She had lost a beloved husband, and a valuable adviser who had stood by her side since the early days of her reign. His death left a void in her life which nothing could ever fill.

The standard of moral purity set by Queen Victoria and Prince Albert was inflexible. It demanded much, especially from people in the public eye, who were expected to set an example in proper conduct. No breath of scandal, no shadow of unconventional or suspicious behavior must ever touch them. No indulgence must ever be shown toward other people's sins, nor could anyone be too strict or too particular about such matters. The private and public life of the royal couple was the living embodiment of a new era in propriety, filial affection, morality, and tranquil domesticity. Prim sobriety, respect for royal and spiritual authority, fidelity to the marriage vows were the hallmarks of the age to which Victoria gave her name.

The least departure from or infringement upon any of these virtues caused her incalculable distress. In her enthusiasm for wifely fidelity, she permitted no divorced lady to come near the court. Indeed, she was even more strict—she severely disapproved of any widow who remarried. This eccentricity may have stemmed from the fact that she herself was the offspring of a widow's second marriage.

So determined was she upon promoting her views of proper morals throughout the breadth of the land that she wrote a letter to the editor of the London *Times* and urged that he "frequently write articles pointing out the immense danger and evil of the wretched frivolity and levity of the views and lives of the Higher Classes," which he did—but five years later.

Her relentless insistence on deference under all circumstances was carried to the extreme. For example, her ministers had to remain standing during audiences with her. On one occasion the prime minister, after recovering from a serious illness, came to consult with her. She remarked that she was sorry she could not ask him to be seated! How different from the behavior of the young queen on the day she came to the throne when she rose and kissed her two elderly uncles to prevent them from kneeling to swear their allegiance to her!

She was remote from the social movements of her time. As the noted English historian, George Macaulay Trevelyan, put it,

"Towards the smallest no less than towards the greatest changes she remained inflexible." The significance for all classes of society of the immense industrial development that was taking place, along with the growth of scientific knowledge, both so well understood by Prince Albert, scarcely touched Queen Victoria.

The agitating atmosphere of reform that stretched over five years, beginning in 1869, aroused her anger and outspoken disapproval. She felt sure that if Albert had been alive, such things would never have happened! But the failure of her protests and complaints served only to intensify her struggles to stem the tides of change that were sweeping across the land.

She found it difficult, and often failed, to distinguish the trivial from the essential, so absorbed was she in a routine that left her only dimly aware of what was happening. Had she realized and properly evaluated the political evolution that was weakening the status of the Crown toward the end of her reign, she would have been filled with extreme displeasure!

Middle-class Britons, proud of their own respectability, rejoiced over their most respectable of queens. She set the tone. They imitated. Many of her characteristics and attitudes were often found among members of the middle class—manners, for instance, which were decidedly aristocratic.

And if Victoria was ill-disposed toward change, a similar reluctance was to be found on the part of many of her subjects, especially when it came to women and the possibility of their assuming a more active, and less housebound, role in society.

In the middle of the nineteenth century in England it was rare indeed for girls to attend most of the schools then in existence. Girls from poor families worked in the textile mills or as domestic servants until they got married. In the middle-class families of merchants, clergymen, landed gentry, and professional men, girls were taught at home by governesses who had some degree of literacy. They were employed to teach reading and writing. At best, they were the meek, ladylike, undereducated daughters of the poorer clergy, or of shopkeepers or mill owners whose businesses had failed.

In the upper classes a governess might instruct her pupils in more than just reading and writing. An advertisement that appeared in the London *Times* in 1845 offered a "comfortable home" but no salary to a young woman who could instruct two little girls "in music, drawing and English." "A thorough knowledge of the French language," continued the ad, "is required."

If primary education for girls depended on the quality of their governesses (when they could be found—and afforded), secondary education for girls was even less available. Families often sacrificed their daughters' advanced schooling in order to pay for the expensive education of their sons. Britain's Education Act of 1870 did provide for primary education, compulsory for all by 1880, but it was not free of payment until 1891. And still, the advantages of higher education were reserved for the sons of the well-born.

Most attitudes toward women in nineteenth-century England were based on a combination of convention, prejudice, and a dislike for disturbance. Among certain groups, there was regard for the finer qualities of women, and fear that if they were to go out into the world and find themselves unsuited to cope with its many pitfalls, they would be wasted, become discouraged, and probably wreck their lives. There was also, however, the possibility that they would rise to the challenge and be able to overcome obstacles and break through barriers erected by society. In that case the danger was even greater. For then they might undersell the men—they would compete with men and might, for example, work for less pay.

The men decided that for girls and women, the "proper sphere" was the home. Men were eager to "protect" women from the "evils of politics." When, after many years of fighting over the right of women to vote, the question came up in Parliament, it was hinted that such a matter was "too sacred to be discussed" in a franchise bill!

As for women's legal status, oddly enough an unmarried woman, at twenty-one years of age, could inherit property and administer it herself without parental control. But when she got married, she became "an infant, legally." Even after she was engaged to marry, she could not dispose of her possessions without her fiancé's approval. After marriage, all her real property, including her personal property as well, and her earnings, if any, became his. She could not, even in her will, bequeath her own personal or other effects without his consent. She could not sue him for divorce, nor could she take legal custody of her children if her husband should divorce her. He had complete right to exercise his authority over her person. He could lock her up. He could compel her to return if she left him. Under the law, she was his possession—a strange contradiction to the marriage vow taken by the groom, who pledged to his bride: "With all my worldly goods I thee endow." In nineteenth-century England, although one woman was queen, most of the others were chattels!

Several humanitarian reforms came about as the result of this century's great social unrest and struggle, but measures to change the quality and quantity of education available for girls were slow in coming. Custom still held back such advantages. It was slow to yield social, economic, legal, or political rights to women.

However, in the economic sphere, England was undergoing an industrialization that was to demand reforms—and very soon. And this growth of the worker population was, in turn, to make the need for reforms in medicine (which had been talked about since the beginning of the century) more pressing than ever.

Textile mills and a variety of industrial and manufacturing enterprises were springing up in cities and towns all over England. In Scotland and Wales, coal mines provided the fuel needed for production in the factories. The working day was very long—in some cases fourteen and sixteen hours—and the pay was very low. More often than not entire families worked in mines, mills, and factories to meet the most elementary needs of life on substandard levels. The schooling of poor children was dependent on what the local parson could do, or could persuade others to do. Fewer than half of England's children attended school, and illiteracy was widespread.

Large numbers of people from rural areas flocked to the cities, or wherever industry was situated, to work in factories, mines, and mills. They lived in overcrowded, unsanitary houses, when they were lucky enough to find such accommodations, and their health was undermined by these conditions and also by the long working days in factories that were just as unsanitary and, as we shall see, were unsafe as well. Coming from the country, as so many did, accustomed to fresh air and sunshine, and used to raising enough, or almost enough, food for their own use, these new city dwellers encountered serious health hazards.

The few hospitals that existed were poorly equipped and poorly staffed. They were not prepared to deal with the accidents that occurred in factories because the moving parts of machinery were exposed. Nor were they able to deal with the epidemics that struck with appalling frequency.

Medical knowledge around the mid-nineteenth century was not great enough to cope with many diseases then prevalent. There were not nearly enough doctors on the staffs of hospitals. Doctors in private practice served only those patients who could afford to pay their fees. And thus the greatest proportion of people most susceptible to breakdown in health—the poor—were excluded from the even limited benefits of medical attention.

Public health—more correctly, the ill health of the public—became a scandal that cried out for some relief.

That relief was offered in the form of the first Public Health Act, and it was passed in August, 1848, effective at once, to run for five years. It provided for a Central Board of Health, with the power to recommend improvements for dealing with public-health matters, but the act did not include a member of Parliament as one of the Board officials (which might thus have made Parliament far more responsive to subsequent needs in medicine). Under this act, local authorities might, but were not compelled, to adopt its provisions, except under certain circumstances. The Public Health Act was adopted by about two hundred localities.

What was it that had finally moved Parliament to acknowledge the need for improved medical care? The most important and compelling reason was that England's second cholera epidemic had gripped London and the rest of the country in 1848. The first cholera epidemic of the nineteenth century struck London in January, 1832. Its ravages had not yet been forgotten by those who had survived it. Can you imagine the terror that hung over crowded, unsanitary, disease-ridden London when the second epidemic hit? The health of the people was, in general, already very poor.

The year 1847 had been marked by a commercial crisis. The poor laws as then drawn did not meet the critical life-and-death needs of the vast number of unemployed and destitute families. Ambitious and greedy manufacturers were sniping away at the Factory Act of 1833, which had attempted to shorten the working day. In 1847, what began as agitation for a Ten Hours Act was soon accompanied by threats of violence and sabotage. But after the big industrialists brought pressure to bear, an act calling for an eleven-hour working day was passed by Parliament.

To summarize the political, economic, and social climate in Britain in 1848, the working day for women and children in textile mills was cut to a hard-won eleven hours. Cholera was stalking the countryside and the overcrowded cities. Of all the local administrative units, only two hundred municipalities, parishes, boroughs—those with a death rate of 23 per 1,000 people—could turn to a local board of health, which, even if it actually had been created and was in operation, could do very little for them. Medical research, such as it was at that time, had not yet been able to isolate the cause of cholera. The doctors were helpless. The death rate soared. People began to lose faith in doctors and in medicine. In a statement that would be amusing if it were not so tragic, the London *Times,* usually favorable to reforms, summed up its bitter opposition to the Board of Health: "[We] would rather take the chance of getting cholera . . . than be bullied into health by the Board!"

The Public Health Act of 1848 was limited, as we have said, to a period of five years. It was renewed for one year in 1853 and finally expired in 1854. The Central Board's most dedicated member was dismissed that year.

The third cholera epidemic broke out in England in 1852, spread through Europe, and struck with great intensity at the armies fighting the Crimean War. A fourth cholera epidemic hit Europe in 1865–1866, and spread to England in 1866. The disease's origin and cause still remained unknown. A very severe outbreak occurred in Egypt in 1883 and caused more than 25,000 deaths. During this epidemic, Robert Koch, the gifted German bacteriologist, discovered and isolated the bacillus that caused cholera. Discovering and isolating the cause of cholera was only the first step. Treatment, cure, and prevention did not come for another ten years!

The reasons for that delay were many. But the most important one was that bacteriology was an infant branch of medicine. Its godfather was Louis Pasteur, whose institute in Paris had opened on November 14, 1888. But he had already been conducting various experiments for several years, some of them aimed at developing vaccines against diseases that were caused by certain specific germs. And here we must remind ourselves that although Edward Jenner had developed a successful vaccine against smallpox in 1798, neither he nor anyone else knew why the vaccination worked.

It was some time before medical curricula in universities added existing knowledge in bacteriology, either as an independent subject or as an integral part of some other branch of medicine. The time lag between developments in scientific knowledge and the integration of that knowledge into medical courses was much too great to enable the new discoveries to play any part in lowering mortality rates. The medical societies, medical faculties, and, in fact, the entire medical profession resisted and even resented the introduction of new methods for the treatment of diseases, or any innovations. Almost all were quite smug and secure in their limited knowledge. The medical profession as a whole was indignant when it became known that some of the most important advances in medical knowledge had been achieved by scientists who were not even doctors of medicine! Indeed, the medical doctors, trained in universities that had not yet incorporated the new discoveries and techniques, usually either could not, or would not, attempt to expand their knowledge when papers dealing with new ideas were read before professional societies. But their deficiencies did not prevent them from deriding or rejecting the ideas as well as the speakers.

As we have said, frequent epidemics, crowded living conditions, faulty and inadequate sanitary conditions, long working hours, and malnutrition all contributed to poor health. It was often necessary to seek medical attention wherever it could be found. Clinics and hospital facilities were limited. Private doctors were costly. And there was nothing to prevent someone from putting out a shingle and calling himself a doctor!

All sorts of quacks promised complete cures for every conceivable disease. Many gave patients medicines they had concocted themselves as part of the miraculous cures they guaranteed, at fees that were low enough to encourage frequent visits.

Medical education was not uniform in content throughout

Britain, nor was it so standardized that all medical students could be required to pass an examination attesting to the fact that the minimum number of medical subjects had been mastered. The public had no way of distinguishing between a quack, especially one with a highly cultivated "bedside manner," and a qualified, competent physician.

In 1856, the *Association Medical Journal* published an analysis of the composition of England's medical profession, listing the physicians' names, their degrees, and where they were trained, as recorded in the *Medical Directory for England* of that year. Following the statistical analysis was an editorial that concluded: "We have shown that at present there is no security whatever [especially for the public], that a man shall have obtained a sound medical education. Around 1500 gentlemen now in general practice have received not one scrap of examination in medicine; while of 800 apothecaries, who, for all we know, are daily engaged in surgical operations, not one has gone through the 'bones'. . . ."

In 1815, an act of Parliament had attempted to legislate some medical reforms, but, the 1856 article stated, "illegal practice has increased most enormously during the last 41 years." It was no wonder that the public was demanding reform, and even from within the medical profession came this confession from the author of the *Association Medical Journal* article: ". . . if any [reforms] were needed, how absolutely necessary. . . . We cannot be worse; therefore, any change must be for the better."

The outcome of public demand that procedures connected with the examining, licensing, and registration of physicians and surgeons be clarified and regulated was the passage of the Medical Reform Act of 1858. It was an admirable bill in several respects, but it made no reference to women.

Before 1858 women were not accepted in British medical schools. They did, however, practice midwifery. But midwifery was not included in the category of medicine, as we have seen.

Some English and other women had studied medicine and had received medical degrees from European universities. But they were not permitted to practice in Britain because the right to practice medicine was granted, under the new Reform Act of 1858, exclusively to students who had completed their studies in a British institution. And in Britain, as we noted, women were not accepted as students in medical schools.

One of the clauses of the new act, however, permitted medical graduates already in practice in 1858 to have their names inscribed in the Medical Register. It was that wedge upon which women based their claim—their right to study and to practice medicine legally in Britain.

It was at this juncture that Elizabeth Blackwell, who had scored such a triumph in America, was to aid the cause of the women in England. She had been practicing for about seven years when she came to England to continue in her profession. Under the entering wedge mentioned above, she claimed—and won— registration in the Medical Register and, therefore, the legal right to practice.

The stunning effect of her action was not lost upon a small group of young women in Britain who had the urge to follow in her footsteps by preparing themselves to serve the sick, especially the women and children, about whose well-being the male doctors seemed to be so inattentive and indifferent.

Just how these five ladies proceeded to fulfill their objectives will be the subject of the next chapter.

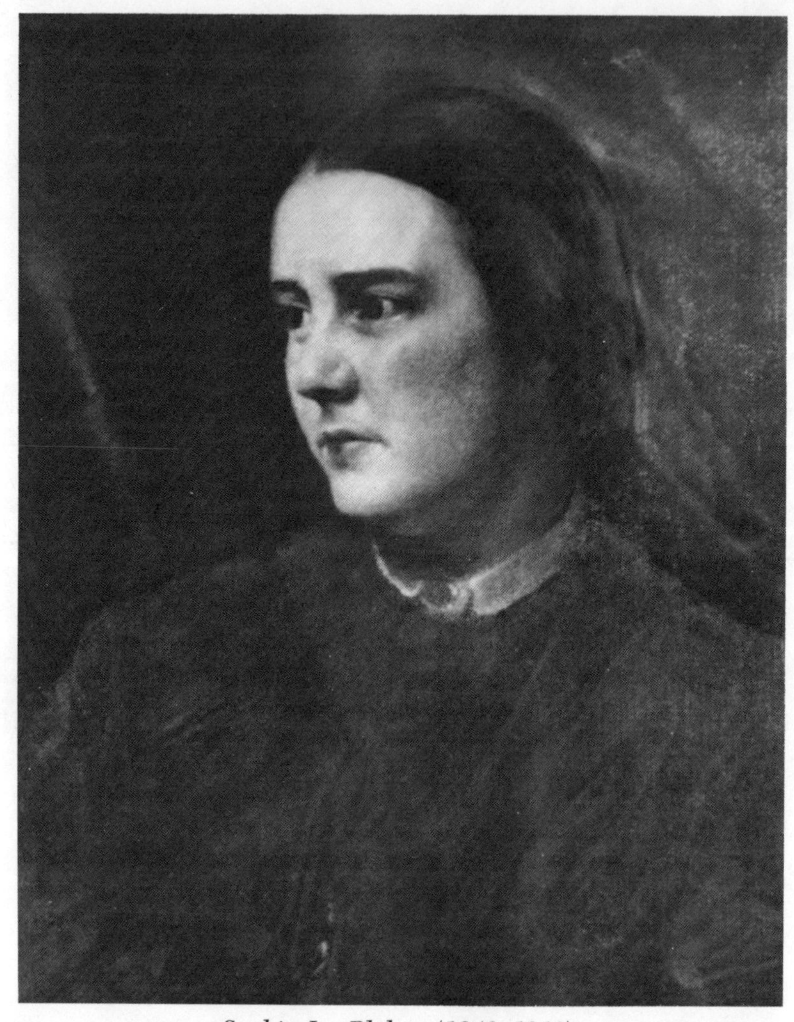

Sophia Jex-Blake (1840–1912)

If Elizabeth Blackwell's success in winning the right to practice medicine in England had been a step forward, the next woman to gain admission to the medical profession was to bring about a serious reversal in this progress.

Elizabeth Garrett (1836–1917) decided in 1860 to study medicine. Under the Medical Reform Act of 1858 there were nineteen institutions that could give medical degrees, and one of these was called Apothecaries Hall. (Actually, not all these institutions had medical schools; some only conducted examinations.) The charter of rules for Apothecaries Hall obliged it to admit any person to take the examinations, provided the conditions of study had been met.

After having been refused by a number of medical schools, Elizabeth Garrett was finally accepted at Apothecaries Hall, but she was not admitted to all the classes with the male students. So she hired private teachers, at great additional cost, for those subjects from which she was barred. After she had completed her studies and, with great difficulty, had managed to complete her hospital training, she took the examinations at Apothecaries Hall and was given a license, which entitled her to be registered in 1865 in the Medical Register as a licentiate of Apothecaries Hall. Here now was the second woman who was ingenious and determined enough to

3.
Sophia Jex-Blake, the "Originator"

overcome the barriers that existed; Elizabeth Garrett thus became the second woman in Britain to outwit the various devices that had been employed to keep women out of the medical profession.

Now the administrative authorities of Apothecaries Hall decided upon drastic action. Feeling that the rules were far too loose, they decided to change them. From that time on, medical students were prohibited from substituting private instruction for class instruction. And so the last remaining loophole was tightly plugged up. A leading medical journal wrote: "We hope that the Court of Examiners [meaning the administrative authorities of Apothecaries Hall] will not stop at this . . . but that they will distinctly refuse to admit any female candidate to examination unless compelled by a legal decision and . . . that they will be supported . . . by [the rest of] the profession. . . ." The new rule definitely closed this and all other doors to any woman who had decided to study medicine in England.

There was one woman, however, who undertook to break out of the cage that held her, and other young, ambitious, and talented women, imprisoned. Her name was Sophia Jex-Blake.

She was born on January 21, 1840. Sophia was the third and youngest child of the family, and her biographer, Dr. Margaret Todd, says that "the home was crying out for a real baby, and all were prepared to treat the newcomer as a little queen." Her childhood reflects that she was ready to live the part. She was vibrant, wholesome, and so happy that in later years, after she was a grown woman whose adult life had been full of strife and battle, she would look back upon her childhood and say: "No one ever had a happier childhood than I."

Though family tradition provided the children with a luxurious home, as a matter of course Sophia's upright and religious parents decided that it would be best for the children if they were denied the social advantages that they themselves had enjoyed. Dancing, the theater, novels, magazines—all were vulgar trash. They looked with favor upon the "mission field" and

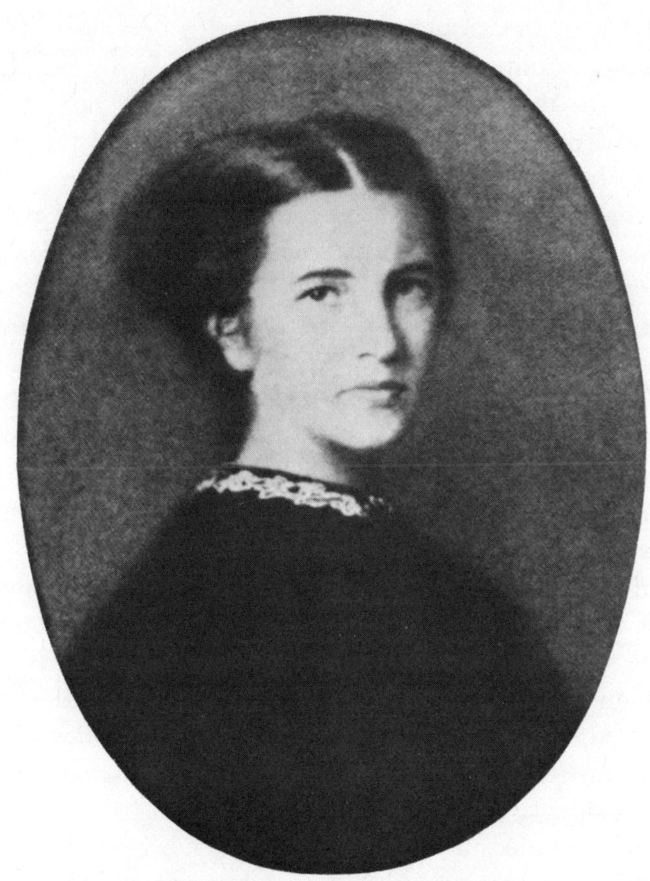

Elizabeth Garrett Anderson   (1836–1917)

encouraged Sophia and her sister to sew small items that could
be sold at bazaars to add to the funds of religious missionaries.
The two elder children fell into this mold quite easily, but not
so Sophia. She was fresh, willful, and naughty, and sometimes
she took her parents' breath away with her pranks. But they
depended on the strong religious influences that surrounded her
to check her outbursts when she would be old enough to understand the consequences of her actions.

She was sent to boarding school with her sister when she was nine years old, after unsuccessful results with education by a governess at home. Her mother's first letter on the day of Sophia's departure admonished her to "overcome self-will . . . strive to be gentle . . . you cannot learn anything . . . till you are obedient and have some self-command . . . do not give needless trouble . . . to anyone . . . try to deserve . . . good opinion." Her friends at school considered her "excessively clever but unfortunately [she] knows it, and makes a point of showing it off upon every occasion. . . ." They described her as "very passionate but very penitent afterwards . . ." and as a girl with "many bad habits but [who] tries . . . to get the better of them . . . rather too fond of her own opinion."

When, at the end of the summer term, the headmistress of the school announced that Sophia must leave, the little girl showed no signs of remorse or humiliation. Some old ladies took care of her until her old schoolmistress agreed to take her back into the school. By the time Sophia was fourteen years old, the school reports became more favorable, much to the delight of her parents. And by the time Sophia was ready for college, she had learned how to win friends and how to keep them. Her life at Queens College, while not entirely free from friction, gave her many hours of pleasure and satisfaction in her work. She excelled in mathematics, languages, history, philosophy, astronomy, and theology. In fact, she was appointed to tutor in mathematics, and she derived a great feeling of independence when her "tutor's money" was added to the allowance she received from her father. But a strong disagreement arose between Sophia and her parents. They wrote that "accepting wages belong[s] to a class beneath you in social standing, and which [friends would say] you had no right under any circumstances, to appropriate to yourself."

"You, Daddy," replied Sophia, "as a man, did your work and received your payment, and no one thought it any degradation, but a fair exchange. Why should the difference of my sex alter the laws of right and honor?" And she continued, "Of course the question of right or wrong, honor or dishonor, is the point. This once settled, people's opinion is worth nothing. I should be glad that my friends had the sense to see clearly and rightly in the matter. If they had not, I regret it for their own sakes,—not for mine." Her father again tried to win her over, but without success. As matters turned out, though, she did give up the fees for the term during which the correspondence with her father took place. But she had her regrets. She called herself a fool, saying she had only deferred the struggle. Sophia was obviously no echo of what her parents and relatives expected. In 1862 she went to Germany and spent some time as an English teacher in Mannheim at the Grand-Ducal Institute, where she evidently met with much success. Needless to say, her parents' efforts to dissuade her, gently but firmly, had no effect.

Can you imagine what a revolution erupted in 1864 when she broached her desire to go to America? The crossing of the Atlantic was a considerable venture for a young woman in those days. To say that her parents regarded the new journey with grave misgivings would be putting it rather mildly. But in 1865 Sophia left for America. Her destination was Boston, where she had a good friend, Dr. Lucy Sewall, a young woman who at that time held the post of Resident Physician to the New England Hospital for Women and Children. (This hospital had been founded in great measure through the efforts of Lucy's father.) Lucy Sewall and Sophia had a warm friendship, and by this means Sophia was introduced to the world of medicine. But even more significant, she came into direct contact with the wider questions surrounding the feminist movement.

In England, the stirrings of women in the feminist movement had been in progress while Sophia was at Queens College, but she had been completely uninterested. The movement was perhaps more subtle at that time. In America it was most explicit; its aims were more clearly defined, of much wider scope, and even partially realized. Sophia began to see the whole world and the part women could play in it if they were not prevented from using their energies and their talents. She was thrilled by her meeting with Ralph Waldo Emerson, the sights of Niagara Falls, and her visits to Oberlin College and Antioch College. She came to know several other women doctors in Boston and even helped out at one of the hospitals there. And now she began to wonder about her own future niche in this wide new world that had been revealed to her. Her good friend Dr. Lucy Sewall had encouraged her to become a doctor, and Sophia's own inclination in that direction had been fanned by what she had observed at Lucy's hospital and by the women doctors she had met there.

In 1866 Sophia began her career in medicine in America, at the New England Hospital for Women and Children in Boston, where excellent work was done in relieving the sick, and where competent doctors were trained. But the medical school facilities existed for men only. Sophia felt that while hospital work such as nursing, carrying out doctors' instructions, etc., was important, nothing could be properly done without an adequate education. Her stay of three years in America convinced her that women doctors were needed and wanted. She was later to say that this experience in America and her acquaintance with the women on the hospital staff helped her decide to devote her life to making medical education available to women. Why not give them a fair chance? On every hand, for example, one heard of the splendid advantages that men were given at Harvard. Why not try there for admission, why not ask? As she wrote to Lucy Sewall, "However good . . . it may be, take notice (if I study at all) I don't mean to graduate at any Woman's College,—on principle, . . . or else for vanity and ambition sake, which is it?" Also, she wanted to stay in the New England area with Lucy Sewall and the others. So Sophia, together with a Miss Susan Dimock, applied for admission to Harvard Medical School.

Harvard replied that there "is no provision for the education of women in any department of this university. Neither the corporation nor the faculty wish to express any opinion as to the right or expediency of the medical education of women, but simply to state the fact that in our school no provision for that purpose has been made, or is at present contemplated."

Now began for Sophia what turned out to be a dress rehearsal for the events that were to follow in Edinburgh just about two years later. She learned a great deal from the next few months. She set about obtaining an introduction to each of the professors on the medical faculty at Harvard and to each member of the staff of the Massachusetts General Hospital and of the Eye and Ear Infirmary, also to others in high places with connections at these and various other institutions. Then she began to canvass them, each one in turn, and asked them for letters expressing their opinion on the matter of medical education for women. One of these important people was Dr. Oliver Wendell Holmes, father of the famous judge. He wrote: "I should not only be willing, but I should be much pleased to lecture to any number of ladies for whom we can find accommodation in the anatomical lecture room." But even so liberal a person could not make his offer unconditional, for he added, "always provided that any special subject which seemed not adapted for an audience of both sexes should be delivered to the male students alone." A professor, writing to Dr. Holmes, was even more emphatic: "Miss Blake who will hand you this note, wishes me to say that I am strongly in favor of the admission of persons of her sex at the Medical College. As such is my decided opinion, I write very willingly." These responses by individual professors did not prevent Harvard from exerting its veto, however. Sophia's comment: "All [of] which ends in . . . smoke! . . . Those wise men of Gotham at the Eye and Ear think it 'the kindest and most gentlemanly thing' to shut us out after all!"

Sophia wrote to Harvard Medical School again, entreating

that they reconsider their policy on the admission of women, but, finally, when "fighting on for Harvard with a sort of dull persistency" held no promise, she gave up Boston in despair and went to New York, where she joined forces with Dr. Elizabeth Blackwell and her sister Emily, both of whom were working out plans for more adequate medical education for women by organizing special classes. Sophia attended those classes, worked very hard at her studies. She had at last found her place in the world and meant to use this opportunity—and her talents—to the fullest. (Miss Dimock, incidentally, went to Zurich to complete her education.)

But then the death of Sophia's father called her back to England. Lucy Sewall did not find it easy to let her go. Her first letter to Sophia was prophetic: "If you don't come back to America, you won't give up the work. You will open the profession to women in England!" And so it came about that Sophia Jex-Blake sought a medical education in her native land. Seasoned fighter that she had become, determined to show the way, she was convinced that she could make this road an easier one for others to take, even the less fortunate, especially the daughters who could not count on as much understanding and help from their parents as she had finally won from her own mother and father. Still Sophia wrote, "I wish very much that I could find some English lady to go in for Medicine with me, it would be such a comfort in thundering at the Colleges, and in working afterwards!" But for the moment she would have to go it alone.

Sophia began by writing to various prominent people for advice on the best way to proceed, and, incidentally, to get their support. She received conflicting answers. Some even suggested that she should go to any one of several European countries where the path was open. But to what end? she asked herself. To gain the right to practice medicine in Britain, she would have to qualify under the Medical Reform Act of 1858. She would have to earn a degree from one of the nineteen institutions listed in that act. Only after getting that degree would she have the right to be listed in the Medical Register. There was no other way. She would have to break through the barriers that existed against admitting women into one of those nineteen institutions.

The registrar of the University of London had made no secret of the fact that the officials of that university had deliberately plotted to exclude women students and prevent them from becoming medical-degree candidates. A friend at the University of Cambridge said, as far as the possibility of admission there was concerned, "I do not think that the most sanguine reformer would advise you to look for any relaxation of barriers that would be of service to you, for some years. . . . I do not think that we will be giving degrees to women until after ten years at least!" Actually, neither Oxford nor Cambridge offered a full medical curriculum in 1869, a further reason to eliminate them from consideration.

And so Sophia turned to Scotland. The Scots had the reputation of taking rather liberal views on policies affecting education. In addition, the Scots boasted that they were free from church-imposed authority and other restraints.

In Scotland the question of excluding women from the study of medicine had never been considered. Scotland had never been faced with the problem. (As you will recall, even though Dr. James Barry had received her degree from the University of Edinburgh in 1812, no one had known that she was a *woman* doctor.)

In seeking admission to the University of Edinburgh, Sophia was really confronting four different groups, all of which might pass on her admission to the university. First, there was the medical faculty itself. Second, there was the Senatus, the university's governing body. It consisted of the university president (called the principal) and the professors of all the faculties in the university. Third, there was the General Council, consisting of those graduates who had registered as its members. Fourth, and finally, there was the University Court, including the influential members of the administration and five other appointed members. The university could, therefore, count on at least four effective guardians against an invasion of women who aspired to be medical students!

By the time Sophia formally applied for admission to the University of Edinburgh it was March, 1869—and Sophia was twenty-nine. For a short time before she had been visiting with each member of the medical faculty and placing her request before them, at the same time asking for their support at the meeting of the medical faculty that was soon to take place to discuss the basic issue—whether or not to admit women as medical students. (Some were on her side, and some were opposed to the admission of women students—violently opposed. One man told Sophia point-blank that he "could not imagine any decent woman wishing to study medicine—as for any *lady*, that was out of the question.")

The foremost opponent among those ranged against Sophia, and against all women who might seek to enter medicine, was Robert Christison. He not only held a very high—in fact the most influential—position at the university, but was also on every one of its ruling bodies. Christison was appointed Physician to the Queen in 1848 and was knighted in 1871. He never at any time wavered in his opposition to medical education for women. He kept insisting that any prohibitions against their admission should remain in force. Even when some of his colleagues had second thoughts on the matter and were prepared to listen to arguments in favor of the young women, he remained adamant. He was convinced that "female practitioners were not wanted in this country . . . that [they] would be injurious to medicine as a scientific profession and that, in the nature of things, the constitution of the female mind and frame is, with rare exceptions, quite unsuited to the exigencies of medical and surgical practice." Ironically, he was not so strongly opposed to women as midwives.

His hostility knew no limits. When he was president of the British Medical Association, he managed to arrange for the exclusion of women from membership. It appears that he used his position as the queen's physician to speak in her name. When an international medical congress was taking place and he was, of course, present, he said he was convinced that the queen's patronage would be withdrawn if women were admitted. And the women were excluded!

His methods were ruthless. According to the wife of one of the Edinburgh professors, Christison threatened to resign if women were admitted to the university. This was a serious threat to the medical faculty and its status in the academic world—and Christison knew it. He was betting his stature in the medical profession and his value to the university against one unknown young girl, hoping to make admitting Sophia or any other woman a policy too costly for the university to pursue.

Sophia, however, was as undaunted as her illustrious opponent was ruthless; she called him "the ogre." He told her during a personal interview that "the matter *has* been decided," and he was "quite uncompromising," saying flatly that he would "use no influence, but vote against [Sophia]." Since he was the only person, as Sophia wrote, "who has all along been a member of every body, without exception, by whom our interests have to be decided, viz., Medical Faculty, Senatus, University Court, University Council, and Infirmary Board [this board was to figure in later battles]," he could not be ignored nor could his position be lightly dismissed.

Then a suggestion was made to Sophia that had some chance of success. Teachers who were friendly to her suggested that she get permission to attend summer classes in botany and natural history. This would prove her competence as a student and her ability to do the work of the entire medical curriculum. While this plan was being discussed in all the administrative bodies of the university—a necessary procedure to obtain permission to

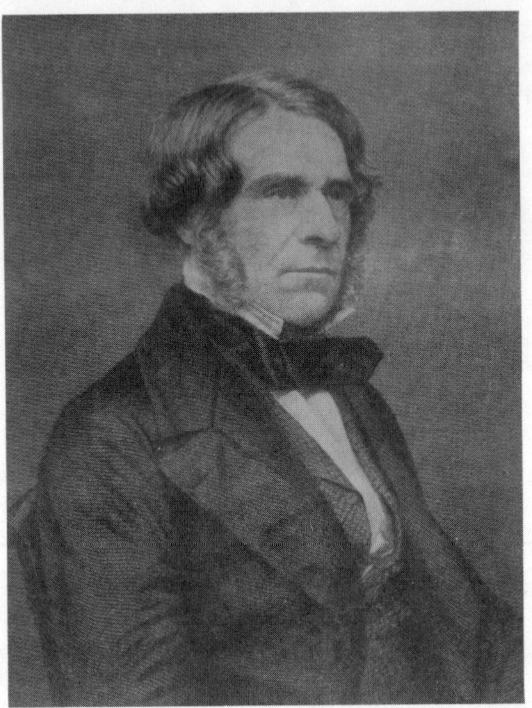

Sir Robert Christison   *(1797–1882)*

attend even those classes—Sophia continued her personal interviews, now with each person who would be involved in voting on her request for that permission. The plan was to do very well in those two subjects and then secure admission to the medical school in October. So she addressed a formal letter to the dean of the medical faculty, basing her request for admission on the fact that the "universities of Paris and Zurich have already been thrown open to women." Sophia writes in her diary: "The thin edge of the wedge in, and, though nothing is secure till after the Senatus on Saturday, yet it is an enormous triumph! . . . If I can be the first woman to open a British University . . . then surely I . . . shall have served, my heart and I—even if I die straightway. . . ."

The opposition of the doctors, everyone said, was the thing to be most feared, and the medical faculty did vote in her favor. True, permission applied to the summer term only. (Possibly some professors were counting on that experience to quench the zeal and spirit of that one solitary woman.) By 10 P.M. on Saturday Sophia was able to record in her diary: "Success—and *such* a success—14 to 4!" Fond of using Latin and French phrases, Sophia then asked herself, *Nunc dimittis?* (Now do you give up?) "No, surely," she answered, "fresh zeal and energy for lifelong work. Isn't it *good* after such a fortnight of rush and battle and strain to go to bed, saying—'The work is done!'"

Sophia became the woman of the moment. Invitations came to lunch and dine with this one and that one. Some of the professors' wives even offered to accompany her to those summer classes if no others came forward.

But the air of optimism was short-lived. Some professors and students, unlike the gallant young men who invited Elizabeth Blackwell to Geneva Medical College, appealed to the University Court against the decision of the Senatus. In April, the University Court met, in secret and in strict privacy, as always. The resolution passed at that meeting stated that "owing to the difficulties at present standing in the way of carrying out the resolution of the Senatus, *as a temporary arrangement in the interest of one lady* . . . [the University Court] sustains the appeals and recalls the resolution of the Senatus."

The newspapers reported this reversal of the earlier favorable decision. *The Scotsman* was in favor of Sophia's cause, and its editor used his columns freely to defend the principle of medical education for women. Other newspapers besides *The Scotsman* were now on the alert for the latest developments on this battle-front. Sophia began to receive all sorts of letters from women who supported her position, and they encouraged her not to falter. "O England," wrote a Mrs. Josephine Butler, "what a wicked amount of conservatism of selfish customs have you to answer for!" And she told Sophia, "I daresay to yourself your life must appear sometimes to be wasted—but it is not so! In every good cause there must be martyrs and pioneers, who, with gifts for more, have had the hard task of opening the way for others to work. . . ."

A letter from a Mrs. Isabel Thorne offered "if you renew your application, [I would like] to join you in doing so, and I believe I know two or three other ladies who would be willing to do the same. . . . I feel a great interest in promoting the entrance of women into the medical profession."

Sophia was joined by Edith Pechey, Mrs. Isabel Thorne, Miss Matilda Chaplin, and Mrs. Helen Evans—as fine a quintet as one could find to undertake to do battle with the formidable power structure of the University of Edinburgh. All through the summer of 1869 Sophia tried her hand at prying open the gates of other universities in Scotland, such as St. Mary's, where she had a good friend in Dr. King Chambers, and the universities in Aberdeen and Glasgow. One by one, all of these possibilities became impossibilities, but she returned to Edinburgh with renewed determination. It now became necessary to arrange for professors who would consent to teach the group of five young women at fees that would make it advisable, from the professors' viewpoint, for them to give up their time. (Fees were at that time paid to the professors and not to the universities.)

Now that a group of five women sought admission, Sophia once again, during that summer, approached the University Court through its president, asking whether they would remove their veto if women could meet in separate classes and, if so, whether these women could then matriculate in the usual way, take the examinations, with a view to obtaining medical degrees. In her usual methodical manner, she also wrote to the Senatus, asking them to recommend the matriculation of women as medical students on the understanding that separate classes would be formed. Next she wrote to the dean of the medical faculty offering on behalf of her fellow students and herself to guarantee whatever minimum fee the faculty might fix as payment for the separate classes. (Her negotiations with various professors had arrived at a figure that amounted to four times the fees paid by the male students.) It is not known what three of the young women replied when Sophia informed them that some such guarantee would add strength to her request; but we do know that Edith Pechey replied, "I am afraid I shall not be able to afford more than double the usual fees for a man."

It was not long after this that Edith Pechey was to write to a favorite aunt about "Miss Jex-Blake the originator of the movement to whom we owe all; and I assure you it requires no ordinary woman to be the prime mover in a movement like this. She must make up her mind to bear rudeness and coarseness from many making high professions of gentility. . . ."

Surprisingly enough, it was from Christison that Sophia had encountered, on the surface at least, just such gentility when she had interviewed him in the course of her efforts to find instructors. He told her, "If anything can be done to get the ladies out of their difficulty, I should be glad to be the one to give them assistance." When that statement was published in *The Scotsman,* its editor added: "The Professor, in spite of his verbal gallantry, has flatly refused either to instruct them himself or facilitate arrangements by which any one can do so in his place."

On July 5, Monday, while her petition for admission was being considered by the University Court, one of Edinburgh's four "guardian" constituents, Sophia wrote, in anticipation of a favorable decision (she was wont to jump the gun when it came to exulting to her diary over potential triumphs): "Even now (4:30 P.M.) a University of Britain may be literally open to women,—if so, won't that have been worth doing?"

And she wrote to Lucy Sewall: "I am working on my Latin, etc., for the Matric. examination. It would astonish the women studying in Boston to see the examination that we have to pass here before we can even begin medicine,—and it is a capital thing, because it will keep out ignorant and silly women to a great degree. . . . I am very glad to see that the British Medical Journal encourages the opening of classes for women. . . . I am only anxious now to have a good class of women and of a creditable kind."

On July 23, the University Court, yielding to public pressure, granted her petition. She was almost too tired to feel jubilant, but she confessed that she would be "grieving bitterly had things been otherwise." Added to all her other work she had been nursing several severe cases of scarlet fever at the house of a friend, since trained nurses for private homes were almost unknown in those days, and she knew it was important to save her strength for the study of Latin for the matriculation examination.

On October 19, the high-spirited little group of five young women made their way to the university to take the preliminary examination in arts (the matriculation examination) which was required of all medical students.

Not only did they all pass, but they passed with grades far above the average. They were all on their mettle; and as one newspaper pointed out, "Out of a crowd of 152 candidates . . . among the seven foremost are four women." Without a doubt, these women were bent on obtaining, in spite of all difficulties, a thorough knowledge of their profession. They were far more thoroughly in earnest than were most of the male students. For that very reason their ultimate success was certain. Another newspaper, reporting their outstanding success, warned that "those who wantonly throw obstacles in the way of this gallant little band incur a proportionately heavy responsibility, as wanting not only in the spirit of chivalry, but even in the love of fair play, which we should be sorry to think wanting in any Briton."

Although the girls had passed the matriculation examination, there was still the problem of arranging classes and, most important, of actually being accepted as students, which meant being granted certificates of admission by the university. Edith Pechey, just taking the first steps toward getting a medical education and, hopefully, becoming a physician, wrote at this time to her aunt:

15 Buccleuch Place
Edinburgh, Oct. 23, 1869

My dearest Aunt,

Your kind letter was most welcome and encouraging coming when it did in the midst of difficulties with professors, etc. I am always glad to get the good wishes of those whose opinions I value, and it pains me extremely when I find that some of those I love cannot agree with me, though I am quite sure that if they thought about it as long and carefully as I have done they would come to see that it is a right and good step. You may be sure if I had not seen it to be not only the right path, but absolutely the path of duty I should not have attempted anything which for the first year at least, will be attended with much disagreeable opposition besides the great dislike I have to doing anything which must bring one at all prominently forward. You will be glad to hear that all our class passed the examination which took place last Tuesday and Wednesday, and I believe I may say I did not disgrace the cause—Our papers I believe were much above the average and we had very good marks in all. Now I think there is less chance of their refusing us admittance. The Council meets in a few days and their decision will do much toward deciding our fate. We have two classes arranged for the first term—physiology and chemistry and we mean to do well in both. I am determined there shall be no handle for opposition on that score. . . .

Ever dearest Aunt, with much love,

Your affectionate niece,
Edith Pechey

We shall soon see whether or not Edith's "doing well" was to be a "handle for opposition." For the moment, however, it was clear that the girls' success on their preliminary exam, as reported in the newspapers, had further intensified public pressure for their admission, and the University Court's resolution granting Sophia's petition for admission was approved by the General Council on October 29, 1869, and by the chancellor of the university on November 12. On that date, regulations drawn up by the University Court were officially issued and published in the university calendar (similar to the catalogue of American universities), where they reappeared annually for the next several years. These regulations stated that

(1) Women shall be admitted to the study of medicine in the University.
(2) The instruction of women for the profession of medicine shall be conducted in separate classes, confined entirely to women.
(3) The Professors of the Faculty of Medicine shall, for this purpose, be permitted to have separate classes for women.
(4) Women not intending to study medicine professionally may be admitted to such of these classes, or to such part of the courses of instruction given to such classes as the University Court may from time to time think fit and approve.
(5) The fee for the full course of instruction in such classes shall be four guineas; but in the event of the number of students proposing to attend any such class being too small to provide a reasonable remuneration at that rate, it shall be in the power of the Professor to make arrangements for a higher fee, subject to the usual sanction of the University Court.

[In 1869, four guineas came to about $21.50, quite a large amount in those days for each course, especially in view of the fact that the male students only paid about $5.00 per course.]

(6) All women attending such classes shall be subject to all the regulations, now or at any future time in force in the University, as to the matriculation of students, their attendance in classes, examinations or otherwise.

(7) The above Regulations shall take effect as from the commencement of session 1869–70.

Consequently, and in accordance with the regulations, the women received their certificates from the dean of the medical faculty, paid the usual fee, inscribed their names in the university album, which committed them to promise obedience to college discipline, and received the usual matriculation tickets bearing their names and declaring them to be *Cives Academiae Edinensis.* They were also registered as students of medicine by the registrar of the Branch Council for Scotland in the Government Register, kept by order of the General Council of Medical Education and Registration in the United Kingdom. (Such registration was obligatory.)

Congratulations were many and came from various people who had closely followed all stages of the struggle. Dr. Elizabeth Blackwell, who had now settled in London, wrote: "It seems to me the grandest success that women have yet achieved in England; it is the great broad principle established that conducts to every noble progress."

An entry in Sophia's diary for a day early that November fairly shouts the news from the hilltops: "The deed of life was done!—This morning, 11:30 A.M. I, S. J.-B., first of all women, matriculated as *Civis Academiae Edinensis!* Tonight for the first time 5 women are undergraduates!— HURRAH!"

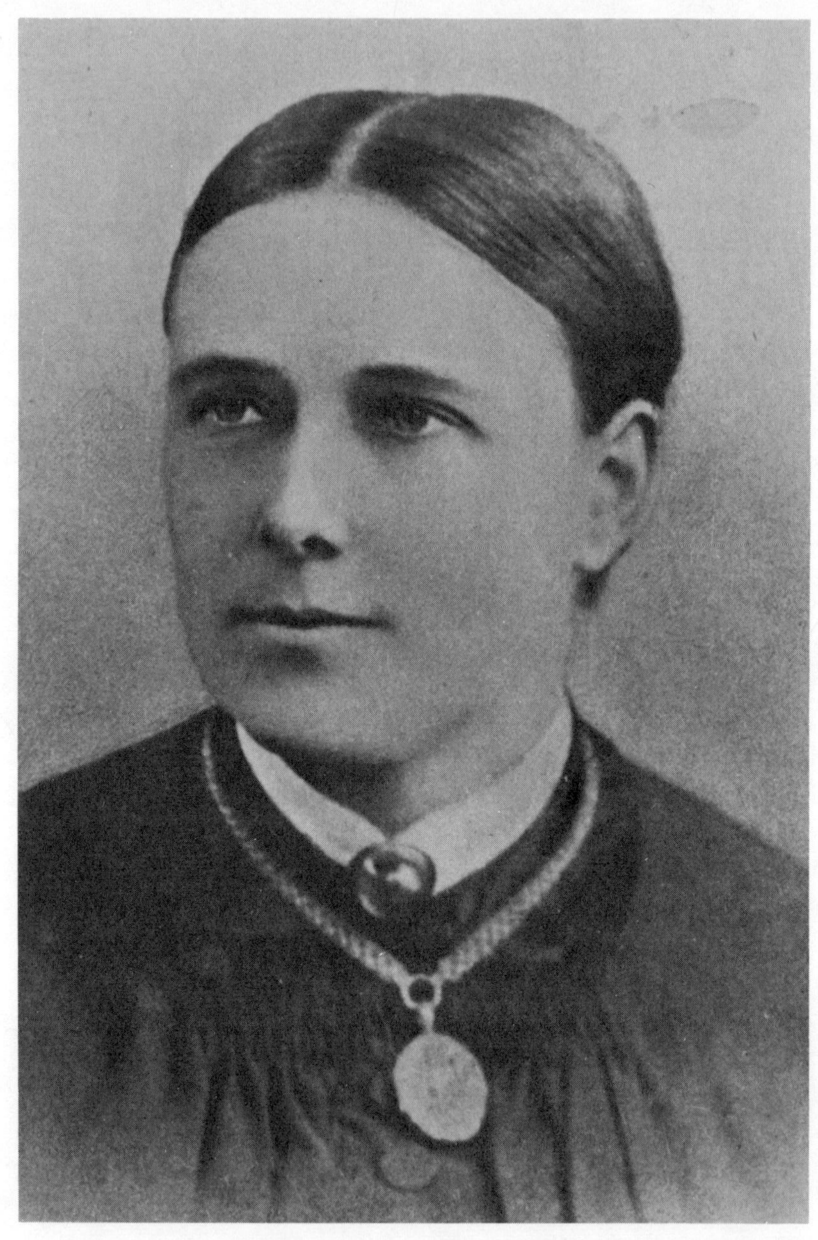

Edith Pechey   *(1845–1908)*

On October 10, 1869, Sophia moved into No. 15 Buccleuch Place, a nice, airy, roomy, wholesome house, at a cost of about £45 in rent, including taxes. Edith Pechey became her roommate and her good strong right hand. They had lunch together the day after Sophia moved in. A week later Sophia described her new comrade in these words: "I think her strong, ready-handed, with 'faculty,' great ability, resolution, judgment; great calmness and quiet of manner and action, and probably strength of feeling; good taste, good manner; very pleasant face; rather good feet and hands; considerable sense of humor; lots of energy and interest in things,—witness dissecting the slugs, keeping caterpillars, etc. In fine, as good an ally and companion as could well be had." As time went on Sophia had more than one occasion to add considerably to this estimate, but never to subtract from it.

Edith was younger, more adaptable, less likely to be alarmed about their future prospects, but even so, possibly more really critical. She was born in Langham, near Colchester, on October 7, 1845, and was the sixth of seven children. Her father was a Baptist minister—in other words, a religious nonconformist in Anglican England. He had been a brilliant student of Greek, Latin, and Hebrew and, ironically enough, had received his M.A. in 1833 from the University of Edinburgh, the very

4.

The "Gallant Little Band" at Edinburgh

same university that was to become a battleground for his daughter and her companions thirty-six years later. Edith's mother was competent in Greek and other subjects, which was extraordinary for a woman in those days.

For a few years Edith taught school. And she also had the experience of being a governess in a rather well-to-do household. Governesses were usually very poorly paid and often worked for food and lodging only, always on call, caring for the spoiled offspring of the rich or middle-class family. For one with a social conscience, this surely was *not* the way to spend one's life! Sophia's crusade offered greater opportunities for self-fulfillment and social service. It is fair to say that Edith saw Sophia's efforts as yielding not only much more education for herself and other women but also as a great benefit for women and children whose health might be improved and whose lives might be saved.

Another factor influencing Edith's decision was that her financial resources were limited. She could not count on much help from her parents. Her father's earnings during the years from 1840 to 1851, when he was the Baptist minister at the small Baptist chapel in Langham, were hardly enough to provide for a family of seven children. By 1869 he no longer held that position. His means must have been very meager indeed. So Edith's decision at the age of twenty-four to undertake at least four years of medical study, for which she would herself have to provide tuition costs and living costs, was a serious commitment on her part.

She realized, too, that it would not do to be just a mediocre student, but that "the first few women who offer themselves as candidates should stand *above* the average of men in their examinations." She put it this way in writing to Sophia: "Before deciding finally to enter the medical profession, I should like to feel sure of success—not on my own account, but I feel that failure now would do harm to the cause. . . . Do you think anything more is requisite to ensure success than moderate abilities and a good share of perseverance? I believe I may lay claim to these, together with a real love of the subjects of study, but as regards any thorough knowledge of those subjects at present, I fear I am deficient in most. I am afraid I should not, without a good deal of previous study, be able to pass the preliminary exam you mention as my knowledge of Latin is small and of Euclid still less. Still, if no very extensive knowledge of these is required (and doctors generally seem to know very little of them) I could perhaps be ready by the next exam, and the study . . . at the same time would be a relaxation."

Mrs. Isabel Thorne came to Edinburgh with a vastly different background. She had spent the early years of her married life in China, where she lost her only child, who, she thought, might have been saved if more skilled medical attention had been available. Doctors in China, as elsewhere, were more interested in and successful with men than with women and children. Mrs. Thorne was convinced that qualified women doctors were badly needed, and when she returned to England, she enrolled in the newly founded Ladies' College for study in chemistry, anatomy, hygiene, and midwifery. She joined Sophia's group soon thereafter.

Little is known of the backgrounds of the other two young women of the Edinburgh quintet, Matilda Chaplin and Mrs. Helen Evans. Matilda Chaplin was twenty-three when she came to Edinburgh, and Mrs. Evans was probably some ten years older. Sophia had first met Helen Evans in the spring of 1869 and had described her as "a very nice woman of 33 or 34 with curiously white hair" and "clear good eyes and face." Sophia found, at their first meeting, that "she and I held together on almost all subjects. She would like to study Medicine (and I am sure has the power). . . ." Mrs. Evans was "much disposed . . . to Botany," but, when she had joined Sophia's group and was pre-

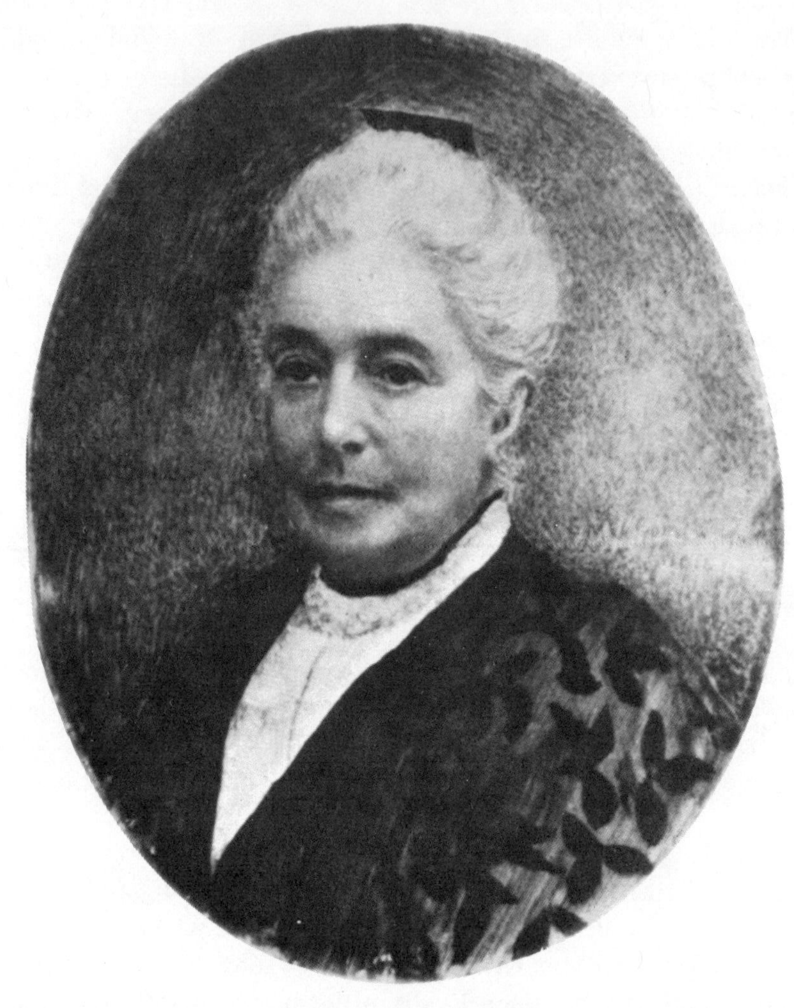

Isabel Thorne (1836–1917)

paring to seek admission to the university, Sophia had to coach her in arithmetic.

Both Mrs. Evans and Mrs. Thorne may have been divorced, or possibly widowed, when they were at Edinburgh, but we do not know for sure. And we don't know precisely how long Mrs. Evans and Matilda Chaplin actually stayed at the university, but we do know that their paths were to be closely linked with Edinburgh for some time.

The house in which Sophia and Edith Pechey lived soon became the meeting place for special little circles. It is hard to decide whether Sophia or Edith was more responsible for drawing them there. Sophia led the group in most matters, but she relied and even depended on Edith more than on any of the others. And if she was a most interesting person to live with, she was by no means an easy person, particularly since she was usually overstrained and overworked. She often gave others advice which she herself did not follow. Her diary on New Year's Eve of 1869 records with truth not unmixed with justifiable pride: "I suppose no such . . . important year in my life. One very dear friend won,—one strong ally,—Edinburgh opened!—What if one *is* a little tired? 'After long travail good repose!' I see that a year ago I thought there were no hopes 'now bright,' and 'an hour of joy I knew not was winging its silent flight.' . . . The year has been glorious in many ways."

Not all the parents and relatives of that handful of students reacted with the encouragement and joy that the events warranted. A mother of one of the young women, when informed that her daughter had received her certificate of formal admission to the university, replied, "Have you?" Her uncle said: "What good is it?" Her sister said: "I am very glad to hear it, but I am very much surprised." But Sophia's family, despite earlier misgivings, was thoroughly sympathetic. Her brother, headmaster at a school for boys, wrote her a long letter; he encouraged her, in terms that would no doubt have appealed to his pupils, to stay,

like a locomotive, on the "medical rails. . . . They are real and
solid and really lead somewhere. . . ." He told her he had felt
for years "and feel increasingly" that "for a large class of delicate
cases, women, when properly trained are the right physicians. . . .
Stick to [the rails], head and hands and feet. . . . Don't be
drawn aside into tempting and irrelevant bye-ways. . . . to have
helped to bring about the result that for years to come girls shall
not be without the pale of professional and University education,—shall not waste their best years in chafing at want of elbow
room at home—will be a great and additional satisfaction. . . .
What you have got to do is to prove that a Lady Physician can
be trustworthy and a success. Do nothing but your work, and you
will do your work well. Of course, get hold of the widest and
deepest Professional education within reach."

There were several difficulties, however, involved in the
newly won victory. For example, professors were not *compelled*
to lecture to the women's class. They could refuse to do so, even
for subjects that the university required. For that first term, the
winter of 1869, five lectures a week in chemistry and in physiology, respectively, were settled. Anatomy lectures and dissections
were still under discussion with the professors. Sophia undertook
to pay one third of the £100 that the anatomy subjects would
cost for the class of five because "two of the students are not
at all rich." "I feel sure," she said, "that one does more good
in thus concentrating one's energies and one's funds to get one
thing done thoroughly than in frittering away lots of small sums
in charity. . . ." She wrote to Lucy Sewall: "It *is* a grand thing
to enter the very first British University ever opened to women,
isn't it?" Her comrades were profuse in their expressions of
gratitude to Sophia for having so persistently worked to win this
precious right for them.

Many professors at the university viewed teaching the five
young women purely as a matter of business. They lectured to
enormous classes of male students, from whom they themselves,

as we have said, collected fees. Why, then, take on additional work for that small group of five women?

An exception was Dr. Crum Brown, professor of chemistry, who was soon to find himself in the middle of the girls' first major battle. He had agreed to teach the young women without hesitation about fees. His reward as a teacher was the high quality of that small group of young women. Edith Pechey in particular, whose interest in chemistry had led her to set up a makeshift laboratory in the quarters she shared with Sophia, where she carried on experiments, became even more intensely engrossed in the subject. The winter session ended in March. So far so good. But now the girls were to learn a bitter lesson about what it really meant to be a woman student here. Edith had done so well that she was first among all the first-year students in chemistry—but when the list of top scholars was made up, her name was placed third on the list, two second-year male students (who had attended the class before) preceding her. What made this not only an injustice but a calamity for Edith was that it denied her the right to receive a Hope Scholarship and the title of "Hope Scholar." The scholarship was actually a £250 prize, awarded to the highest-ranking first-year student in chemistry, and with it went the privilege of having free access to the college laboratory. Can you imagine what that scholarship would have meant to Edith Pechey? The money was badly needed, but the free access to the laboratory quite likely meant even more to her. She was first among all the first-year students, male and female, no one denied it. But by proving her outstanding ability in chemistry the very first year she studied the subject, she stunned the already hostile professors and also the many prejudiced male students, who could not accept this evidence of female mental excellence. As one of the women's ardent supporters said at this time, "A woman must have uncommon sweetness of disposition and manners to be *forgiven* for possessing superior talents and acquirements!"

Brown tried to get himself out of an awkward position by explaining, rather lamely, that Edith, having studied at a different hour from the men, was not a member of the official chemistry class. So he issued the women written certificates stating that they had attended "a ladies' class in the University," but he was only getting himself into deeper trouble, for these were worthless and would not be accepted for credit when it came time to take the professional examinations and show that proper study in chemistry had been completed.

The newspapers and even a leading medical journal let loose a howl of indignation over the whole country when the story of the chemistry prize became known. Professor Brown, despite his friendly help to the women and the high quality of his teaching, was singled out for attack both inside and outside the university and rather unjustly became the administration's scapegoat.

Brown certainly bore the women no grudge. In his own way he was the friend and helper of their struggling cause. After all, when Sophia had first approached him about securing his services as a teacher, he had written, "I am convinced that the experiment [of admitting women] must be made. . . . I therefore cordially agree to your proposal." But Brown had been in Dresden when he had sent this reply to Sophia. Now he was back in Edinburgh, where the climate—especially the academic climate—was different. It is even possible that Brown was ordered by the administration to see that Edith did not receive the scholarship; nonetheless, he did award Edith the official bronze medal of the university, and it could be claimed only by a member of the chemistry class. And he put her name and names of her companions in their rightful places on the published honors list. What a clumsy—but well-intentioned—compromise!

The Senatus was consulted in the matter, and, by a majority of one, they decided that Edith Pechey was not entitled to the Hope Scholarship and, also by a majority of one, that the five women *should* have the regular class certificates.

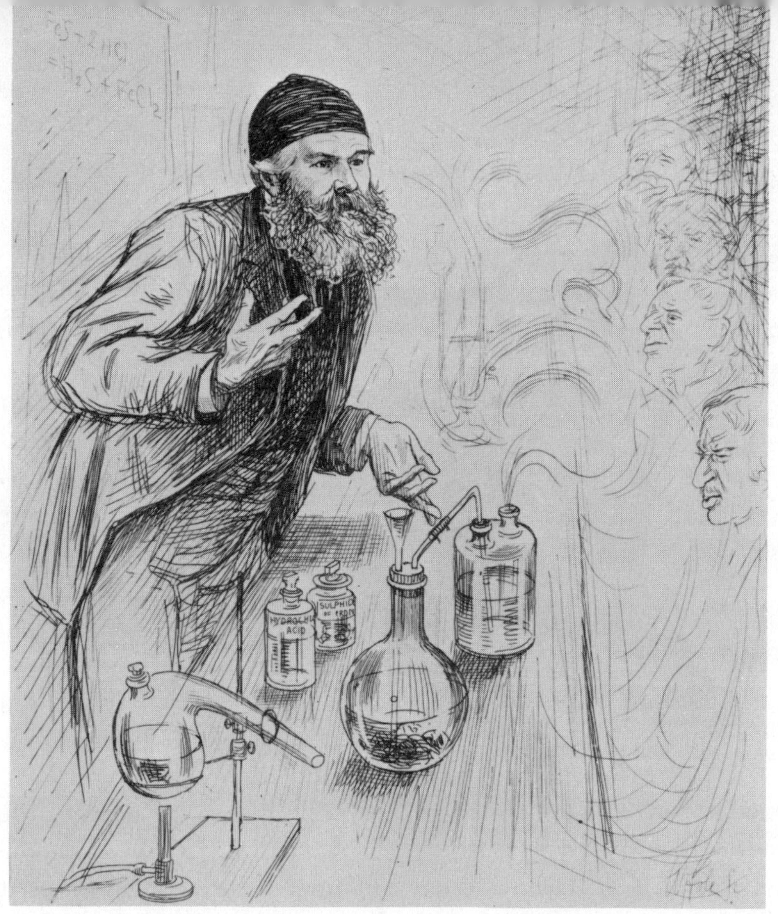

Professor Alexander Crum Brown (1838–1922)

Dean Masson explained the apparent contradiction to Sophia in this letter: "I agree with you that the one vote stultifies the other and I think people are seeing this. At the time I made up my mind that the first vote must carry the other unfavourably with it; but it was not for me to keep the Senatus consistent, and when [Professor P. G. Tait] announced his view, I grasped at the unexpected accident and seconded his motion."

The outcry continued, because the general public knew little or nothing about differences between one certificate and another, but they knew what it meant to lose a scholarship! Again a leading medical journal spoke its mind quite sharply: "Whatever may be our views regarding the desirability of ladies studying medicine, the University of Edinburgh professed to open its gate to them on equal terms with the other students; and, unless some better excuse be forthcoming in explanation of the decision of the Senatus, we cannot help thinking that the University has done no less an injustice to itself than to one of its most distinguished students."

In the lives of these women, one dilemma after another became almost an everyday occurrence. They weighed the advisability of appealing the Hope Scholarship matter to the University Court. Edith had gone home to the country, and she wrote to Sophia: "I wish you were here to tell me what to do. You understand that I leave you to do as is thought best about the scholarship,—only remember that my own judgment—apart from personal feeling—is against appealing, and that I do not wish to do so unless our friends are very decisively of the opinion that we ought to." And so the matter was dropped.

If Christison was the women's implacable enemy, and Brown their somewhat hesitant but friendly "helper," the dean of the medical faculty, as a result of the scholarship case, had become their firm friend. Dean Masson had come to the conclusion that one of the basic problems (and what had led in large part to the whole scholarship imbroglio) was the fact that the women were taught in separate classes. He sought to remedy that arrangement, and presented a motion to this effect at the next meeting of the General Council of the university.

Once again a matter that one might expect to stay well within the university walls was taken up by the newspapers. Opponents of the resolution were vehemently indignant and had used language so abusive that the *Times*, although it disapproved of mixed classes, sharply rebuked Christison and a certain Professor Laycock in its lead editorial: "We cannot sufficiently express the indignation with which we read such language, and we must say that it is the strongest argument against the admission of young ladies to the Edinburgh medical classes, that they would attend the lectures of Professors capable of talking in this strain."

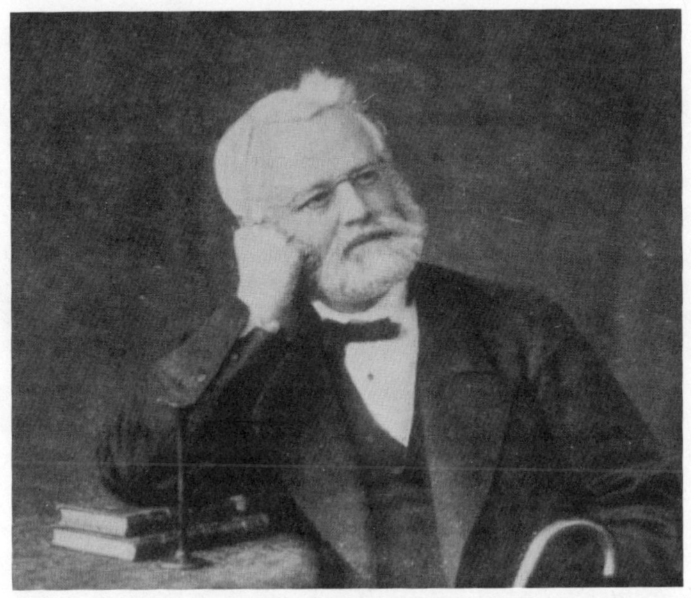

Thomas Laycock (*1812–1876*)

Despite Dean Masson's efforts the motion for mixed classes was not carried. The *Spectator*, another of the newspapers joining in the fray, deplored the "concessions" thus made to "English prudery, concessions not made either in France, Austria, or the United States." "Science is of no sex," they said, "and cannot be indelicate unless made so. . . ."

Some years earlier this was exactly what Elizabeth Blackwell had stood up for—but in America she had won. Her anatomy professor had asked her one day to skip his lecture on a "delicate subject." When she wrote him a note objecting to such squeamishness over a "scientific pursuit," the truth came out—it seems that this subject had indeed been made somewhat "indelicate" by the professor's customary inclusion in this lecture of some dirty jokes. The professor admitted his shame over his former conduct, and Elizabeth was invited into the lecture room. She was given a standing ovation; and never again was there any question about her attendance at all lectures on all subjects.

But such immediate victories were not to be won in Great Britain. Dean Masson, in particular, was terribly downcast about the failure of his motion to admit the women to mixed classes. He wrote this detailed report to Sophia:

No speaking on our side could have changed the vote, those present were all predetermined. Crum Brown did well, and administered a proper reproof to L[aycock]. . . . People today are consoling me—for I was really downcast—by saying the result was a success in its kind, and an omen of final success when the thing comes up again, as it must. All very well; but how shall I console *you?* . . . . What shall I say but that my heart is sore for your immediate discomfiture? Time—a year or two—will rectify the thing generally, here and elsewhere; but how you are to get on with us is the question. Christison, who draws Turner, Lister, and Sanders (L[aycock] is nothing) with him, seems determined to get rid of you, and trusts to effecting this by mere continuance of the present arrangement. Whether you can wriggle on with us by any ingenuity in the hope of beating him is for your consideration. Would it might be so!

Ever yours truly,
David Masson

But Edith Pechey, for one, was enjoying the situation, having a good time, and not making a fuss.

Writing to Sophia from her home in the spring of 1870, she admitted that she was very "vexed about the General Council, but it's no use worrying,—at least so the nightingale tells me. She sang two hours at my bedroom window last night, and said all sorts of pretty things. I wish I could bring her to Edinburgh with me, but she wouldn't like it; besides they are a very old family, and have lived in the place from the time of the Britons, so she wouldn't like to move. . . . If the truth were told, [Papa] still has some lurking prejudice against mixed classes. He isn't a bit scientific; never notices the butterflies and beetles in a walk unless I point them out to him, and there are lovely ones now, peacocks and brimstones and tortoise shells."

When the time came for the women to engage professors to continue their courses, Alleyne Nicholson, a professor of natural history, offered to teach them in a summer course provided his students did not object. An affirmative reply came not only from a majority, but from the entire class! And so the first mixed class was introduced. It continued throughout the summer without the slightest difficulty.

Professor Nicholson was a teacher in what was known as the Extra-Mural School and was not on the staff of the university proper. It seems that some years before, students had begun taking these "extramural" classes (classes which met outside the university buildings), which were taught by nonfaculty members, in order to supplement the poor instruction they were receiving in some courses taught at the university. After many years of battling over the practice, the university had finally agreed that four such extramural classes might be allowed to count toward graduation.

In admitting the women to his extramural class in zoology, Professor Nicholson declared: "The course of lectures on Zoology which I am now delivering to a mixed class is identically the same as the course which I delivered last winter in my ordinary class of male students. I have not hitherto emasculated my lectures in any way whatever, nor have I the smallest intention of so doing. In so acting, I am guided by the firm conviction that little stress is to be laid on the purity and modesty of those who find themselves able to extract food for improper feelings from such a purely scientific subject as zoology, however freely handled. 'To the pure all things are pure.'"

So far, so good. Now the really great difficulty was to obtain a professor—one recognized by the university—who would teach the women anatomy and clinical practice. As usual, there were representatives of the university who were not in favor of making that matter easy. One after another the professors refused. In one case, the fees had actually been paid when the lecturer, after much negotiation, finally agreed to teach the class. But soon after, he backed out and returned the fee and apologized. Some who wanted to help had become unpopular with their colleagues because of other unpopular causes they had previously supported, so they dared not take on another and jeopardize themselves and their status still further. Some others, having already agreed because they did not believe the difficulties were real, had to give up when confronted with an opposition that was as impenetrable as an iron wall and could not be overcome.

Professor Turner—in the Christison camp—refused to teach his subject, anatomy, not only to a mixed class but not even to the women in a separate class. Nor would he allow his assistant to teach them. Then, the only extramural teacher of anatomy, Dr. Handyside, stepped in and taught a mixed class when the school term resumed in October, 1870.

Some unfriendly busybody informed the Senatus that the mixed classes in the Extra-Mural School were technically an infringement of university regulations, but fortunately this attempt to outlaw the classes was unsuccessful. Sophia, jubilant with every little step forward in the war the women were waging, believed that mixed classes would be established in the university before the next year, 1871. She wanted desperately to see the future in such an optimistic light because it would then not be crucial each term for the women to plead with reluctant professors to agree to teach them.

But some progress was being made on other fronts. At the October matriculation examinations of 1870, three young women were present seeking enrollment. The examiners were not sparing in their praise of the results these newcomers scored. Here are just a few of their comments: "Miss Barker's logic paper, the best ever had from medical students." "Miss Bovell's French best in

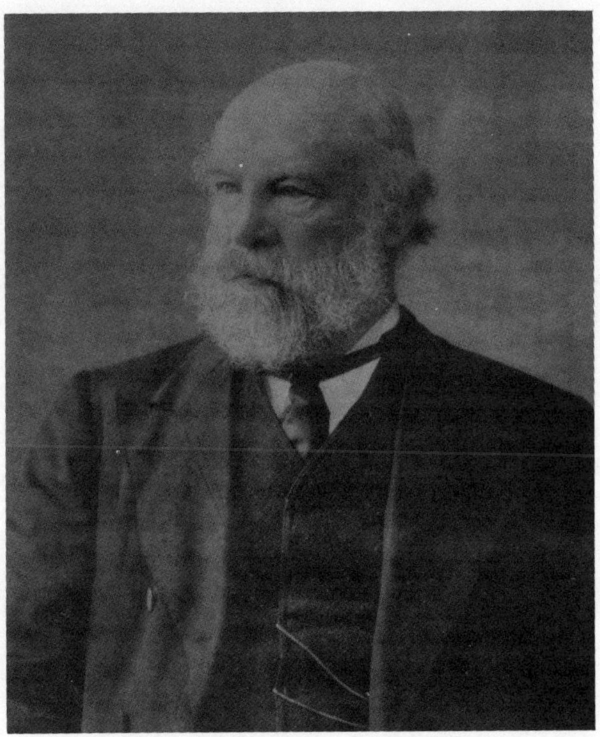

Sir William Turner   (*1832–1916*)

the University, except one Frenchman's." "Miss Walker had the *only* 100 per cent in Mathematics." Unquestionably a triumph for the new women students, this success may have also served to deepen the resentment already felt by many of the men. Women had been at Edinburgh for a year now, and the students were more sharply divided than ever in their attitudes toward them. Though the hostile students usually made the headlines, there were friends as well, and those who were friendly had become more so. Those who had been hostile became (with the prodding of some unscrupulous professors) even more violent in their opposition. Life at the university was not going to be easy for the women this year.

Dr. Handyside's mixed class in anatomy and dissection met in Surgeons' Hall on the main street of Edinburgh. The girls worked diligently and without outward interference, at first. In fact, Dr. Handyside was especially pleased because the male students were more serious than usual about their work, and he commented that better work had never been done in his classroom. Officially, the anatomy class was to begin in November, but the rooms were open and the teachers were present from the beginning of October. The women took advantage of the extra time in those rooms. The male students who did likewise were those who were the most serious about their work, and, consequently, all went about their work in earnest. The women would gladly have welcomed a separate room, but none was available; so they worked away steadily and quietly in their corner, oblivious to everything but their studies.

Then, as now, hospital training was mandatory for all medical students, and the women were advised at this time to apply for permission to work in the Royal Infirmary, the only hospital in Edinburgh large enough to meet the requirements of the General Medical Council for registration as a physician.

Along with her studies, then, Sophia would have to negotiate with the Managers of the Royal Infirmary. An entry in Sophia's diary for November 4, 1870, gives us some idea of what her day was like:

> Just put down this day's work for a specimen! Studying and canvassing at once!
> 8.45. Started for Surgeons' Hall
> 9–10. Tutorial class, bones.
> 10–11. Surgery lecture.
> 11–1. Dissecting.
> 1–2. Anatomy lecture.
> 2.10. Reached home and found a letter from Mr. Blyth (Manager) [possibly a Manager of the Royal Infirmary] telling me to meet him at 2 P.M.! Got there

> (after bolting beef-tea and wine) at 2.45. Talked with
> him for nearly an hour with good results, I believe.
> Got back home 3.40. Bolted some food, and went
> 4 P.M. Demonstration exam. Didn't know the Acromion
> [the part of the scapula at the outer end of the
> shoulder] but got 13/20 marks.
> Home to dinner.
> 7 P.M. Started on round of calls.
> Home at 10 P.M. Not tired,—oh, dear no!

The effort on the part of the women to obtain permission to work in the Royal Infirmary spurred the hostile students, with the overt and covert incitement of some professors, to make a concerted effort to get rid of them. They shut doors in the faces of the women. They crowded into seats usually occupied by the women. They burst into howls and horselaughs whenever the women came into sight "as if a conspiracy had been formed to make our position as uncomfortable as might be," said Sophia.

The students began circulating a petition to bar the women from the Infirmary, and, five hundred students having signed it, they and the rest were prodded to "follow it up. . . . Don't stop there. While you are at it, why not get rid of the women altogether?" With advice such as this, the instigators, including some of the professors, fanned the men's prankish instincts. For a day or two, feeble efforts were made to keep the women out of the classroom in anatomy. Sophia and her companions, looking straight ahead, walked right through.

And then, in a burst of perverted "enthusiasm," on Friday, November 18, 1870, according to *The Courant,* "shortly before four o'clock, the hour when the ladies arrive at the College, nearly 200 students assembled in front of the gate leading to [Surgeon's Hall]. . . ." Even this newspaper, unfriendly to the women's cause, felt constrained to recount the following details: "Shortly before four o'clock those on the outlook descried the approach of the ladies, and immediately their appearance was greeted with a howl which might have made those who are supposed to be possessed of more temerity, quail, but it seemingly had no effect upon the ladies, for they most unconcernedly advanced towards the gate, the students opening up their ranks to allow them to pass. On reaching the gate it was closed in their face. Amidst the derisive laughter which followed this very questionable action, it must be said to their credit that a number of students cried 'shame.' In a short time the janitor succeeded in opening one leaf of the gate, and the ladies were admitted to the precincts, but not before some of them had been considerably jostled.

"The anatomical class-room to which they proceeded was crowded to the door, and, in consequence of the noise and interruption, Dr. Handyside found it utterly impossible to begin his demonstrations. With much difficulty, he singled out those students belonging to his class, and, turning the others out of the room, he was about to proceed, when the pet sheep which grazes at the College was introduced to the room, a student jocularly remarking that it would be a good subject for anatomical purposes. Poor 'Mailie' was kept a prisoner, and the lecturer was allowed to proceed.

"When the class broke up, a number of the students seemed determined to accompany the ladies home; but the result was that several of them were apprehended by the police."

In Sophia's words: "As soon as we came in sight of the gates, we found a dense mob filling up the roadway in front of them, comprising some dozen of the lowest class of our fellow-students at Surgeons' Hall, with many more of the same class from the University, a certain number of street rowdies, and some hundreds of gaping spectators, who took no particular part in the matter. Not a single policeman was visible, though the crowd was sufficient to stop all traffic for about an hour. We walked straight up to the gates, which remained open until we came within a

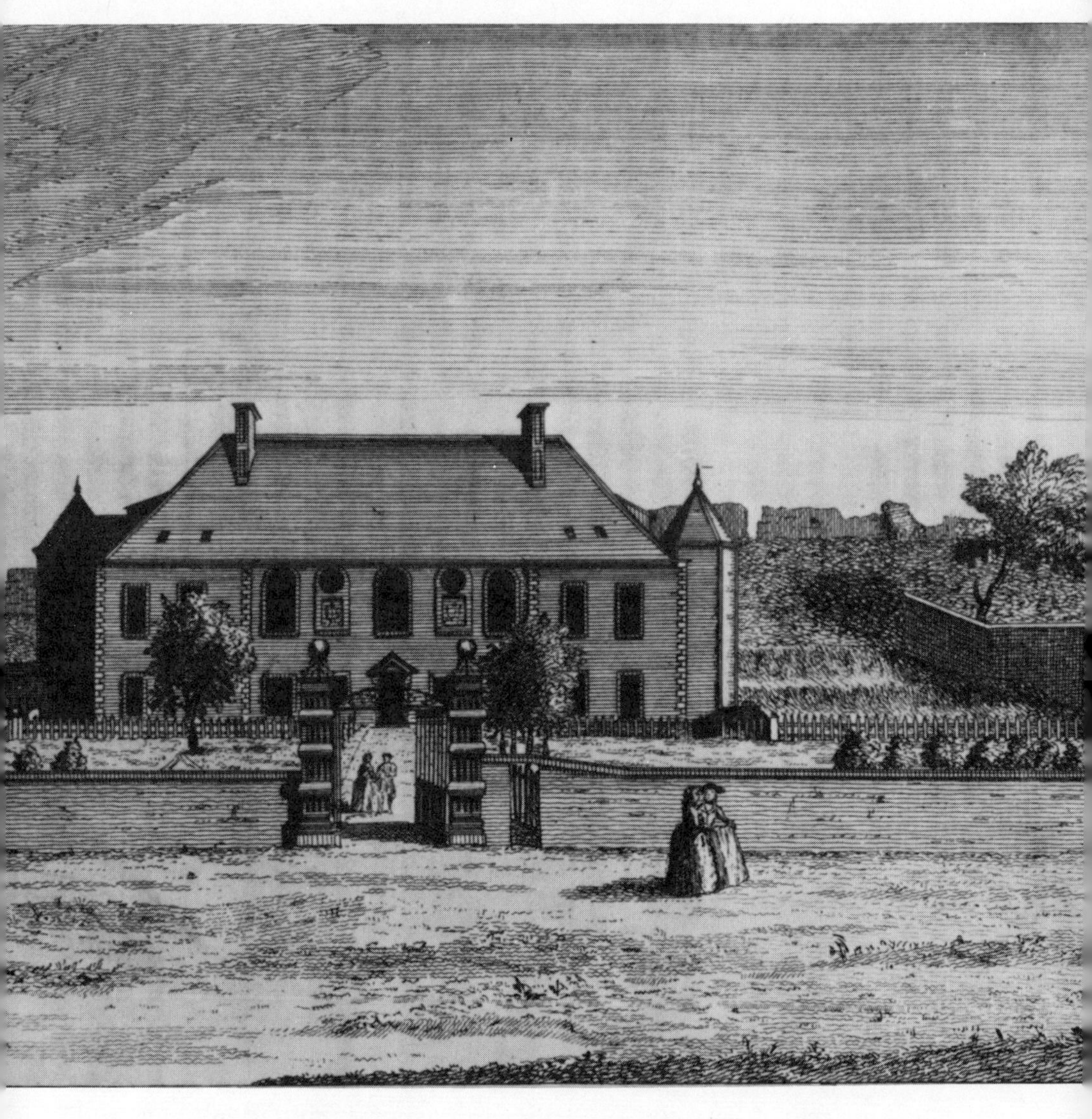

A perspective view of Surgeon's Hall

yard of them, when they were slammed in our faces by a number of young men who stood within, smoking and passing about bottles of whisky, while they abused us in the foulest possible language, which I am thankful to say I have never heard equalled before or since. We waited quietly on the step to see if the rowdies were to have it all their own way, and in a minute we saw another fellow-student of ours, Mr. Sanderson, rush down from Surgeons' Hall and wrench open the gate, in spite of the howls and efforts of our half-tipsy opponents. We were quick to seize the chance offered, and in a very few seconds we had all passed through the gate, and entered the anatomical class-room, where the usual examination was conducted in spite of the yells and howls resounding outside, and the forcible intrusion of a luckless sheep, that was pushed inside by the rioters. 'Let it remain,' said Dr. Handyside, 'it has more sense than those who sent it here.' At the close of the class the lecturer offered to let us out by a back door, but I glanced round the ranks of our fellow-students and remarked that I thought there were enough gentlemen here to prevent any harm to us. I had judged rightly. In a moment a couple of dozen students came down from the benches, headed by Mr. Sanderson, Mr. Hogan, Mr. Macleod, and Mr. Lyon, formed themselves into a regular bodyguard in front, behind, and on each side, and encompassed by them, we passed through the still howling crowd at the gate, and reached home with no other injuries than those inflicted on our dresses by the mud hurled at us by our chivalrous foes. Wilson [a friendly student] came up and took Mrs. K[ingsley]'s arm (to our momentary fright) [Mrs. Kingsley, though not a degree student, had sat in on the class with the others], and we were escorted home by (a) gallant cavaliers, (b) police, (c) general mob, (d) all boys and girls of the town."

On the Sunday following Friday's riot, Robert Wilson, the same student mentioned by Sophia, sent a letter to Edith Pechey: "I wish to warn you, and, through you, your friends, that you are to be mobbed again on Monday. A regular conspiracy has been, I fear, set on foot for that purpose. I wish you to tell your friends that although the projected demonstration against you on Monday is intended to be much more serious than the one on Friday, and to frighten you all away, you need not in the least fear it. I have made what I hope to be efficient arrangements for your protection. I have passed the word round amongst a lot of my friends—not wholly inexperienced in the kind of work —and you will be all right.

"I had a meeting with my friend, Micky O'Halloran who is leader of a formidable band, known as the 'Irish Brigade,' and he has consented to tell off a detachment of his set for duty on Monday. Mickey was the formidable hero with the big red moustache who stood by us on Friday and whose presence with us rather disappointed the rioters who, I think, calculated on the aid both of himself and his set. I have taken care of *that*, and I believe the mere demonstration of the fact that you have men on your side able and willing to protect you, will deter the mob from even an attempt at a row.

"They are a cowardly lot, nearly all very young, and I don't think they have even one amongst them who has had experience of the days when street-rioting was one of the accomplishments Edinburgh students were acquainted with, so they are not likely to be very troublesome. I believe they'll 'cave in' if you only show a brave front. . . . However, as I tell you, you and your friends need not fear, as far as Monday is concerned. You will be taken care of."

On Monday the 21st came another warning of a "more serious demonstration," so Wilson swore in the Irish Brigade. But it rained that day and there was almost no crowd. On Tuesday the 22nd the Irish Brigade—some thirty or forty men— escorted the women home. One townswoman hissed as they passed. Someone in the crowd said, loud enough to be heard by all, "You know they'd never do it if they could get married."

To which someone else answered, "Eh, you're wrong there, there are some very good-looking ones among them." O'Halloran, of the Irish Brigade, escorted Edith Pechey, called her *ma belle*, declared that "a loife wasn't much, but all the Irishmen would lay down theirs before allowing [the women] to come to any harm." Then he shook Sophia's hand till it nearly came off and assured her that it would give him much pleasure to be of service.

The following day the ladies also had their Brigade escort, but according to Sophia it was now "little necessary."

The newspapers printed letters and articles of abuse against the students, and some took a stand against the women. *The Scotsman,* whose strong support of the women consistently brought to public attention the difficulties they managed to overcome, on this occasion not only accused the students, the majority of whom "conducted themselves in a most contemptible manner," but also pointed up the "influence of the classroom where their respected professor meanly takes advantage of his position as their teacher to elicit their mirth and applause, to arouse their jealousy and opposition, by directing unmanly innuendoes at the lady students."

Wilson, the student who had written the women that warning letter, had said he believed that "the real cause of the riots is the way some of the professors run you down in their lectures. They never lose a chance of stirring up hatred against you. For all I know they may have more knowledge of the riotous conspiracy than most people fancy."

The Scotsman asserted, in addition, that the students were "roused not by a word or look from the ladies, but by the possibility of being outstripped by them in the race for honors; and therefore did they elect to end the rivalry by an appeal to brute force. The truth, however, is that the rioters were called together by a missive, circulated by the students in the Chemistry Class of the University, on Friday morning. . . . This missive called

upon the petitioners [those who had petitioned the Royal Infirmary against the admission of female students] to assemble at
the College of Surgeons before 4 o'clock, for the purposes which
they so thoroughly carried out. . . . What is now to be done with
this vexed question of female education?"

Indeed that was the question being asked in many quarters,
for news of the riot had gone around the whole world. Even
Edinburgh's standing as a center of education was challenged as
a result. Though some newspaper accounts were favorable toward
the women and some were not, they did manage to rouse a great
deal of support for the five young ladies at Edinburgh.

"Well," wrote Sophia, "we are about in the deepest waters
now,—that's one comfort!"

But the fight for the Royal Infirmary was still ahead.

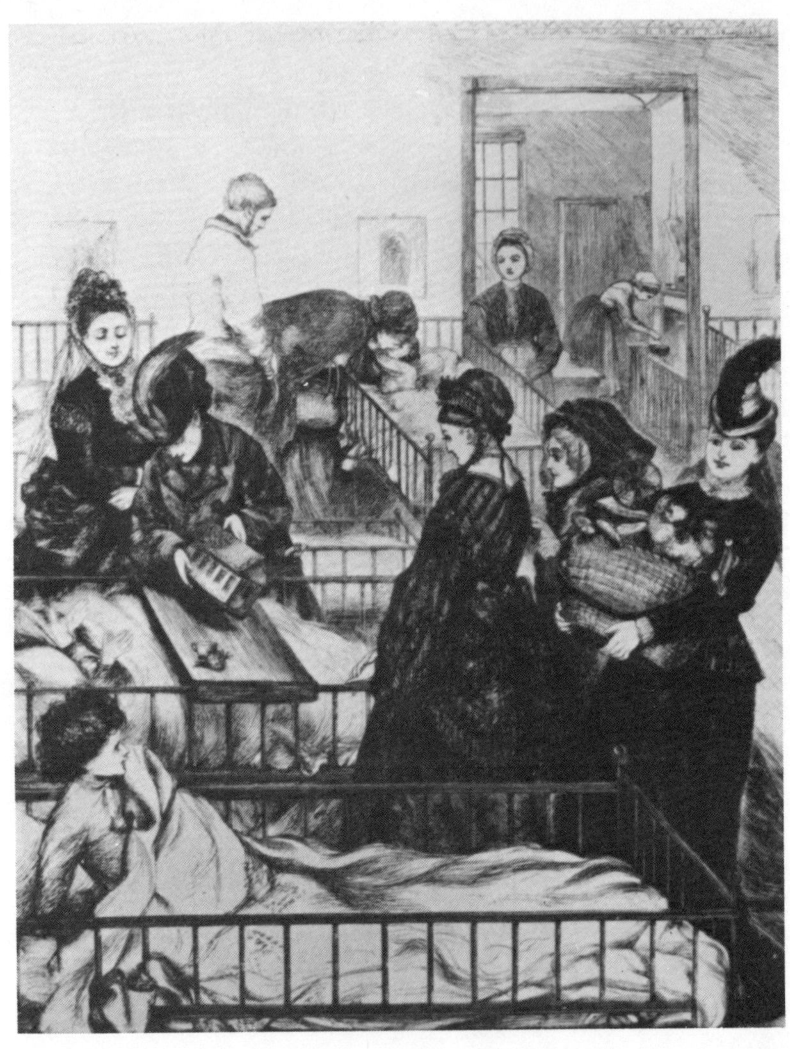

Children's Hospital, Christmas 1869

Sophia and her group were entitled to admission to the Royal Infirmary as matriculated students of Edinburgh University, but their application to the Infirmary, as we have seen, had prompted a petition, signed by five hundred students, asking the hospital to deny admission to the young women; and this, in turn, had led to the riot at Surgeons' Hall.

The Infirmary did deny admission; the refusal was abrupt, blunt, and definitive.

Friendly doctors thought that the hospital charter compelled them to admit all medical students, and they suggested a written appeal in the form of a petition. All of the women students signed a petition stating their intention to work in the wards of only those physicians who consented to instruct them, and to refrain from even visiting the wards of those who objected to their presence as students. The doctors who agreed to instruct them wrote a letter saying that the presence of the women would in no way interfere "with the full discharge of our duties towards our patients and other students." Two others were ready to teach the female students separately "if suitable arrangements could be made in the wards."

The decision now rested in the hands of the Royal Infirmary Managers; as it turned out, an election to choose the next year's Managers was about to be held, so

5.

The Fight for the Royal Infirmary

everything hinged on the election of men who would be favorable to the women's cause. The election was to take place at the Annual Meeting of Contributors (more or less like a meeting of stockholders), which was to be held on January 2, 1871.

The meeting hall was crowded long before the session was to begin, and in fact there were so many people that the hall could not hold them all and the meeting was moved to St. Giles Cathedral, a rather lofty setting for the squabbling and commotion that was about to occur.

To begin with, the official head of the city, the Lord Provost, proposed the election of six men known to be in favor of the women students; but that entire slate was defeated. Then the Infirmary medical staff submitted its slate. Interruptions and heated arguments filled the cathedral. Sophia asked for permission to speak. (She had deliberately become a contributor to the hospital, which entitled her to vote, so that she might speak at this particular meeting.)

She became more and more nervous as her turn approached. Overworked, tired, resentful of the way some in authority were inciting the students to make trouble, she was determined to tell the contributors the whole truth of the unfair attacks upon her and her comrades in their efforts to carry on their medical studies. If the slate of Managers in favor of the women's cause had been defeated, Sophia would at least have her say.

Describing the events that had preceded the riot, she said: During a period of five weeks, the conduct of the students with whom we had been associated in Surgeons' Hall, in the most trying of all our studies, that of Practical Anatomy, had been quiet, respectful, and in every way inoffensive. They had evidentally accepted our presence there, in earnest silent work, as a matter of course. Dr. Handyside . . . assured me that . . . he had never had a month of such quiet earnest work as since we entered his rooms. But at a certain meeting of the managers when our memorial was presented, a majority of those present were,

I understand, in favor of immediately admitting us to the Infirmary. The minority alleged want of due notice of the question, and succeeded in obtaining an adjournment.

"What means were used in the interim I cannot say, or what influence was brought to bear; but I do know that from that day the conduct of the students was utterly changed, that those who had hitherto been quiet and courteous became impertinent and offensive, and at last came the day of that disgraceful riot, when the college gates were shut in our faces and our little band bespattered with mud from head to foot."

"Shame!" cried some in the audience.

Sophia continued: "It is true that other students who were too manly to dance as puppets on such ignoble strings, came indignantly to our rescue, that by them the gates were wrenched open and we were protected in our return to our homes. . . . I will not say that the rioters were acting under orders, but neither can I disbelieve what I was told by indignant gentlemen in the medical class—that this disgraceful scene would never have happened, nor would the petition have been got up at the same time, had it not been clearly understood that our opponents needed a weapon at the Infirmary Board. This I do know, that the riot was not wholly or mainly due to the students at Surgeons' Hall. I know that Dr. Christison's class assistant was one of the leading rioters—"

The audience hissed at this, but was called to order.

"—and the foul language he used could only be excused on the supposition I heard that he was intoxicated. I do not say that Dr. Christison knew of or sanctioned his presence, but I do say that I think he would not have been there, had he thought the doctor would have strongly objected to his presence."

Dr. Christison broke in at this point, addressing the Lord Provost: "I must appeal to you, my Lord. I think the language used regarding my assistant is language that no one is entitled to use at such an assembly as this—"

"Hear!" cried someone in the audience.

"—where a gentleman is not here to defend himself, and to say whether it be true or not. I do not know whether it is true or not, but I do know my assistant as a thorough gentleman, otherwise he never would be my assistant; and I appeal to you again, my Lord, whether language such as this is to be allowed in the mouth of any person. I am perfectly sure there is not one gentleman in the whole assembly who would have used such language in regard to an absentee."

Sophia: If Dr. Christison prefers—

Dr. Christison: I wish nothing but that this foul language shall be put to an end to.

The Lord Provost: I do not know what the foul language is. She merely said that in her opinion—

Dr. Christison: In her opinion the gentleman was intoxicated.

Sophia: I did not say he was intoxicated. I said I was told he was.

The Lord Provost: Withdraw the word "intoxicated."

Sophia: I said it was the only excuse for his conduct. If Dr. Christison prefers that I should say he used the language when sober, I will withdraw the other supposition.

The audience laughed.

Later on in the meeting when Sophia rose to speak again, she had to pay the penalty for having described the students as "puppets." They started to shout, yell, and throw peas at her. Finally, after this stormy episode, the slate of Managers opposed to the women was elected.

Sophia received many letters after this meeting, a number of them expressing regret over the events that had taken place. "I am ashamed of my sex," one man (a doctor) had said. A Mrs. Nichols, who had spoken up at the meeting in favor of the women, wrote to Sophia: "I cannot help feeling that the discussion is doing so much to educate people's minds that it is better for the cause than if you had met with no opposition; and in the end it may be better for you also, for by the time you are ready to practice, persons will have become accustomed to the idea and ready for you."

Sophia's brother sent birthday greetings (she was thirty-one): "One line to wish you many happy returns of the 21st, and most of them quieter than this birthday seems likely to be. I feel sure you will carry your point eventually, and should recommend you to stick to Edinburgh where you have already so very nearly won! . . . I feel no doubt whatever of the ultimate victory, but the delay is very fatiguing to the combatant. . . . Take it easy, and don't let the enemy make you angry. They are sure to try."

The end was not in sight. Both sides were firm. Hospital instruction was lost for that year. The silver lining of that dark cloud, however, was the Lord Provost, who could not accept defeat. He called a meeting of leading citizens of Edinburgh where the groundwork was laid for a committee to ease the burden that had now become far too heavy for the handful of women to shoulder. Committee sympathizers rallied to the cause and became an example for others to follow all over the world. At the first public meeting on April 19, 1871, the name "Committee for Securing Complete Medical Education to Women in Edinburgh" was adopted.

And this committee was to prove quite important to Sophia, for the outcome of that Royal Infirmary meeting had been not the loss of hospital training only but also this—Dr. Christison's assistant, Mr. Craig, was suing Sophia for libel.

It must have seemed to Sophia that this was the last straw! The public meetings connected with hospital admission and the newspaper criticism of her conduct there brought her spirits to their very lowest point. It took no more than a day or two for the whole country to know that her impulsiveness had plunged the little group, and especially Sophia, into a head-on collision with the law and that she would, for the first time, have to be on the defensive side of the case.

Sophia's brother offered to pay half of the legal expenses.

He advised her that it was "vital that you should have the best legal assistance, and win." She herself felt she had nothing to hide and hoped actually to gain from having the opportunity to justify herself and her cause in an open court of law. With public opinion in general opposed to her, and all sorts of rumors in the air, she expected that she would set the lies at rest and win over some of the opponents.

It was at this time that Sophia received an invitation to speak at a meeting of women suffragists in London. Despite her mother's objections, Sophia spoke at the meeting, and she was a great success; for the rest of her life she was to be one of the most practical interpreters of the movement for women's rights.

The days leading up to the trial were not easy ones for Sophia and her four friends. They had gone to the students, hoping to find some support among them. Sophia complained of "the obstinate lying of these students in preference to giving any information possibly useful to us." And in the streets, the women met with "constant hisses and rudeness . . . incivility, insolence . . . shouting 'whore' . . . in George Square Gardens yesterday evening, when one of the group crossed the street."

There were a few "friends and helpers"—a student named Gilbert, and Robert Wilson, the one who had written them the warning letter. The trial was set for Tuesday, and Sophia was anxious to get it over with. "Oh, dear," she wrote, "I hope Tuesday at least will end one worry satisfactorily. I think it must clear me morally at any rate!—and yet I have that nervous quiver through me as when one wakes with a nightmare!"

The case lasted two days. The courtroom was crowded all day both days. Many women were in the audience, and many saw these amazing young ladies for the very first time. One newspaper wrote: "Mrs. Thorne succeeded as witness and the assembled public thought it very hard that she should be neither odd nor eccentric. Why was she married? She was a medical student and ought not to be married! Sedate, quiet and ladylike-looking, and dressed in an unobtrusive fashion, and yet fairly within the pale of orthodoxy, Mrs. Thorne confused the minds of many.

"Miss Pechey . . . created a good deal of fresh interest. A tall figure and a classically shaped head with dark hair, are generally supposed to be the attributes of young ladies who keep to their 'sphere.' That female medical students should dare to be good-looking, dare to be married, dare to be dressed in good taste, is, of course, an unpardonable crime.

"Great interest of course was manifested in Miss Jex-Blake's appearance in the witness box. Plainly dressed in black, with white around her neck and wrists, she presented the appearance of a tall and well-formed, handsome and determined woman, with dark hair and eyes. She was perfectly cool and collected, and her manner was a great contrast to the nervousness of Dr. Christison and the 'smartness' of Dr. Bell."

The case was handled in a rather strange—some people might have said prejudiced—way by a judge selected by the plaintiff, Mr. Craig. Sophia was at a particular disadvantage because she didn't know Craig by sight. She had only repeated hearsay but looked forward to being able "to prove the young man's real conduct in the matter." However, the judge prevented witnesses from answering any questions that would have placed Craig on the scene, and in fact overruled all the objections of Sophia's counsel. Craig had the advantage of a brilliant lawyer, who, in fact, did not even call him to the witness stand, pointing out that Craig "was not so fond of public appearances as the defendant"; the courtroom laughed at this.

Although Sophia appeared to the casual observer to be cool and collected, she must have been in a state of near torture. The "substantial truth and right" which she had looked forward to revealing she never got a chance to tell. The case was full of contention and argument, and whenever Sophia's counsel attempted to bring a relevant fact to the attention of the court and jury, Craig's counsel, Shand, would shout his objections, which the judge almost invariably sustained. To top it all off, the jury's verdict was apparently given without a full understanding of what was involved. They agreed to decide in favor of Mr. Craig, but to award him only one farthing in damages—thus actually making a compromise decision that, if not wholly satisfactory to Sophia's side, did not at least unduly favor Craig's side either. But the jury, as one of its members later explained, had no idea that despite its verdict, Sophia could be forced to pay all of Craig's expenses involved in the suit. She was, and this amount came to almost £1000!

The whole affair, thought some, was a terrible miscarriage of justice, and some people urged Sophia to appeal, but she did not do so.

Contemporary reports gave the distinct impression that the case was conducted so as to arouse hostility toward the women and to damage their standing in the community. As far as the university was concerned, this appeared to have been accomplished. Edith Pechey, though modest and self-effacing as a rule, spoke out in the columns of *The Scotsman* about the "hint" the court's decision appeared to have given to the Edinburgh medical students: "They have been told pretty plainly that it is possible that there should be a riot got up for the express purpose of insulting women, for one of the very women insulted to be accused of libel when she complains of such conduct, and then for the insulters to escape scot-free, and the complainer to be mulcted in expenses. In fact the moral seems to be that, unless a woman is willing to be saddled with costs to the amount of several hundred pounds, she had better resolve to submit to every kind of insult, without even allowing herself to mention the facts. . . .

"It will possibly strike some people as sufficiently extraordinary that a knot of young men should find pleasure in following a woman through the streets, and should take advantage of her being alone to shout after her all the foulest epithets in their voluminous vocabulary of abuse; yet such is the case." She wrote of how "the other night" some students had followed her through the street, "using medical terms to make the disgusting purport of their language more intelligible to me."

But, she said, "each fresh insult is an additional incentive to finish the work begun. I began the study of medicine merely from personal motives; now I am also impelled by the desire to remove women from the care of such young ruffians." Edith had come a long way since she had refused to appeal because the nightingales advised against it.

If the libel case had resulted in worse treatment for the young women at the hands of the medical students, it had yielded some positive results as well. *The Glasgow Herald,* in commenting on the case, declared that the trial had "established nothing," and that "Miss Jex-Blake has completely vindicated the title of her sex to aspire to the highest honors not merely in medicine but in law."

And the entire chain of events—the ugly riot, the denial of hospital training, the obvious injustice in the proceedings during the libel trial, and its outrageous verdict—had made the women's cause a matter of widespread interest, the subject of endless discussions. One of the well-known women of the day, Harriet Martineau, sent a donation to the fund that was set up by the Committee for Securing Complete Medical Education to Women in Edinburgh, and so did Charles Darwin and Thomas Henry Huxley. But such notables were not the only ones to make contributions. A post-office order for eight shillings came from "a few working men" who deeply sympathized with Sophia in her noble "strugle" for the right of women to "a liberal education and remunerative employment." They added their wishes that she be "of good cheer, of good courage, and continue steadfast unto the end." At a public meeting attended by many influential citizens, Sophia was presented with a check for £1000, and after all expenses were paid £112 remained, so Sophia asked that it be added to a fund that she had already been accumulating for the purpose of founding a hospital for women, to be staffed by women.

And so, for the moment, things returned to normal. The women attended a botany class in the summer of 1871, and, not surprisingly, the names of three of the five appeared on the prize list. This summer was to see some good changes taking place. Dr. Lucy Sewall, Sophia's friend from America, was coming to Scotland, and Sophia wrote her in anticipation of that visit: "People are getting wild for women doctors here,—and you might make almost any income, and do quite incalculable good by living here for the next five years. . . . This morning I had a quite spontaneous offer of £200 to help found a Women's Hospital here, and I believe that in a week I could get ten times that amount promised."

But the university professors were another matter. Sophia had complained to Lucy Sewall that "we have eleven women studying here now, and absolutely no one to give them [adequate] uterine teaching." Once again, as the autumn term faced the young women, certain professors—Dr. Christison among them— refused to teach them the required courses. By special arrangements, however—and the payment of extra fees—they were able to secure professors willing to teach them so that they could continue their studies.

That autumn unexpected support came from another quarter. Three more women applied for admission to the university. Edinburgh was not a university to let anything happen easily, and from time to time there was a rumor that an effort would be made to prevent any new women candidates from taking the matriculation examinations that October. And a new crisis was developing. It was rumored that Sophia and the others of the quintet might not be allowed to take the First Professional Examination, a test covering the first two years of medical study;

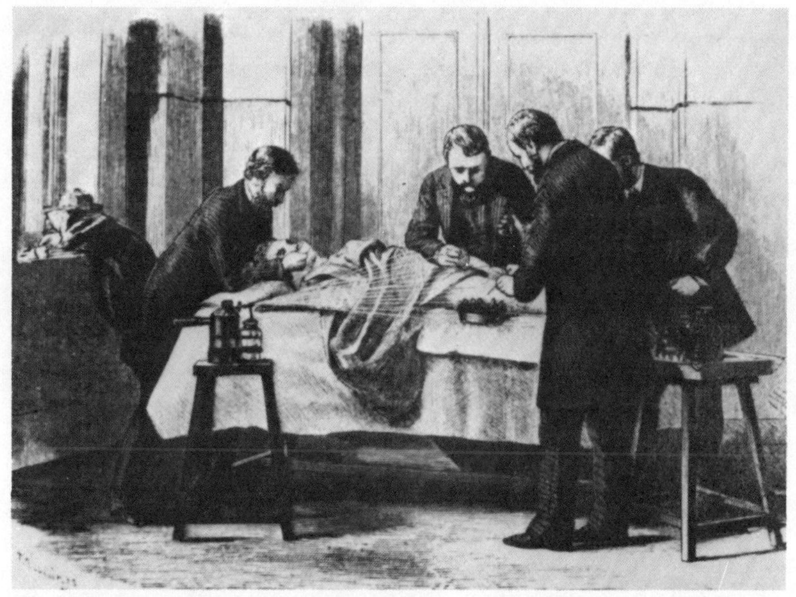

A surgical operation being performed around 1870. In front of the patient is a steam apparatus giving off a carbolic spray to create an antiseptic atmosphere.

this exam was also scheduled for October and was the very goal toward which all their studying so far had been aimed. Once again the women's opponents had found an opportunity to throw up another obstacle. Sooner or later, they thought, we will tire the women out, force them to give up in defeat. But the gallant little band was not so easily defeated. As ever, it was Sophia to the rescue. She consulted with a lawyer and then threatened the university with legal action if examinations were denied either group of women. For once the law was on Sophia's side—and apparently the Senatus knew it, for all the women were admitted to their respective examinations, which they all passed in good order.

But such easy victories were not to be won often. Nine

thousand women from all over England signed a petition asking that the university allow these women to complete their studies, and they presented it to the University Council. A resolution embodying that petition was offered to the Council, and was so vehemently opposed by Christison, among others, that it was tabled.

It seemed as though nothing had been settled at all in regard to this "vexed question of female education," for despite earlier official university rulings admitting the women to the university, the fundamental decisions were being challenged all over again. The newspapers and medical journals joined in, *The Lancet,* the foremost British medical journal, charging Edinburgh with first admitting the ladies and then stopping them "half-way in their career."

Opposition reached such height that in November of 1871 a professor at a meeting of the Senatus urged it to rescind the regulations for the admission of women to the university, but to preserve the rights of those already studying. This proposal was passed by a majority of one. Fortunately, the University Court did not see the issues in quite the same light and declined to put this resolution into effect—but only on the grounds that it was "inexpedient at present" to do so.

At the end of the 1871 winter session the prize lists again carried the women's names, but it was obvious by now that such success was not going to win their opponents over.

They did have by this time, however, some notable champions. Robert Louis Stevenson was one of many still writing and talking about the women. (A relative of his had been one of the "Honorary Treasurers" of the fund raised to pay Sophia's lawsuit expenses.) Stevenson wrote to that relative, Louisa, praising the women as "first of a noble army, pioneers, Columbusses and all that . . . ," at the same time saying that he would not care to marry Miss Jex-Blake or any of her friends in the group. "Let posterity marry them. If posterity gets hold of this letter,

I shall probably be burnt in effigy by some Royal Female College of Surgeons of the future."

But they would not have to wait for posterity to marry them. Despite all the turmoil, there had been time for courtship, and three of Edinburgh's young ladies had married in the past six months. The first to marry was a woman student named Mary Anderson, who, though not a member of the original quintet, had since come to Edinburgh to join the cause. And then Alexander Russel, the friendly editor of *The Scotsman,* came to Sophia one day and told her that the ranks of women students were going to be "thinning" even more. Sophia, reluctant to lose yet another young lady, asked who it was she would be losing. Mrs. Evans, he said.

"I don't believe it!" said Sophia.

"Well, she told me so herself," he replied.

"*Did* she?—and who on earth to?"

He became quite embarrassed, his face got red: "Have you no idea?"

"No," she said, fibbing by this time.

"Really, no idea?" he persisted.

"How should I?"

"Well,—she asked *me* to tell you about it,—does *that* give you an idea?"

"*Mr. R.!* You don't mean to say it's *you?*"

Now he got even redder! "Yes, I do!"

"Well!!!!—I hope your treachery will go between you and your sleep!"

"Now don't you be hard on her! Will you go and see her?" he asked.

"No, certainly not! The most she can expect is that I don't send a policeman after her!"

"And brand her with D?" [presumably, Deserter]

"Yes! You may tell her I won't do that—that's the utmost she can expect!" As Sophia was leaving, she muttered: "Well,

I think you're an uncommonly lucky man, but I hope your conscience will prevent your sleeping!"

And as if this were not bad enough, a month or so later, Matilda Chaplin married one of the university professors— William Edward Ayrton, who was also her cousin.

Sophia received a letter at this time from a woman who urged, "I do hope you and Miss Pechey will remain firm to the end, for really three marriages within six months is quite alarming!"

No, Sophia would never forsake the cause, and she never married. She had become quite a celebrity, and in Edinburgh coachdrivers would tell their passengers, "Miss Jex-Blake had that house last year!" Though her name was mentioned on the stage, in games, and had been in the press for years, she still refused to be interviewed. The public had no idea of the more human side of her character. Her holidays were spent in absolute retirement except for the company of the most intimate of friends.

With Edith Pechey's beauty and charm, it is fairly certain that she was more than once urged to forsake the good fight and the thankless right to be a doctor in exchange for marriage. A scrap of a love letter from an unidentified admirer has somehow turned up. There is no certainty as to whom it was intended for, but it is not unlikely that it was addressed to Edith: "When I came into the anatomical room and saw you sitting there dissecting, I was overpowered, utterly conquered. When I spoke to you and you looked up at me to answer, the look you gave me was the *coup de mort!*—I determined then in my own mind to seek you for my wife. . . . But to see you there with your superlative beauty, working so bravely, so sensibly,—all fashion, frivolity and folly cast aside,—was to me so new, so strange and so admirable a sight, that on considering and re-considering it, I don't wonder at myself for flinging aside ordinary prudence to make a snatch at a jewel of such unusual brilliancy."

It is quite disappointing to reflect that the recipient of this tribute was not equally prepared for "flinging aside ordinary prudence." However often she was urged, Edith Pechey did not marry until eighteen years later—during a most significant period of her life and in another part of the world. Meanwhile, she was deeply committed to the hourly and daily struggles of the women students of Edinburgh. She deplored those events that placed her in the public eye, yet never shrank from her part in those struggles. Their goal was so simple, and single—a medical degree and registration in the General Medical Council's Register.

The immediate problem was still how to gain admission to the Royal Infirmary for training in the wards. The Infirmary, which, as we know, had already once refused to admit the women, was now again about to hold its annual meeting. This time a slate of men favorable to the women was elected; and it was resolved that all registered medical students would be admitted to the educational advantages of the Infirmary without distinction of sex. A heartening shower of congratulations reached the women students after this victory. But their opponents were not ready to give up so easily. They fastened on a technicality of the voting procedure, and, in spite of whatever public support had rallied round the women, their opponents managed to contest their admission to the Royal Infirmary for a full year. When the Managers who favored them finally met to vote formally for the admission of the women, their terms of office had but two weeks to run!

The vote to admit the women was not without limitations. They were restricted to classes separate from the men, and to those wards where the physicians and surgeons would formally accept them. In actual practice, this limited them to about eighty beds, less than a sixth of the Infirmary's total. Yet the objective of admission for hospital training had at last been achieved. And to further that training they found some allies. Dean Balfour, a surgeon, gave them three hours of instruction every week. Dr. Peel Ritchie, a prominent surgeon, gave up a class of men to

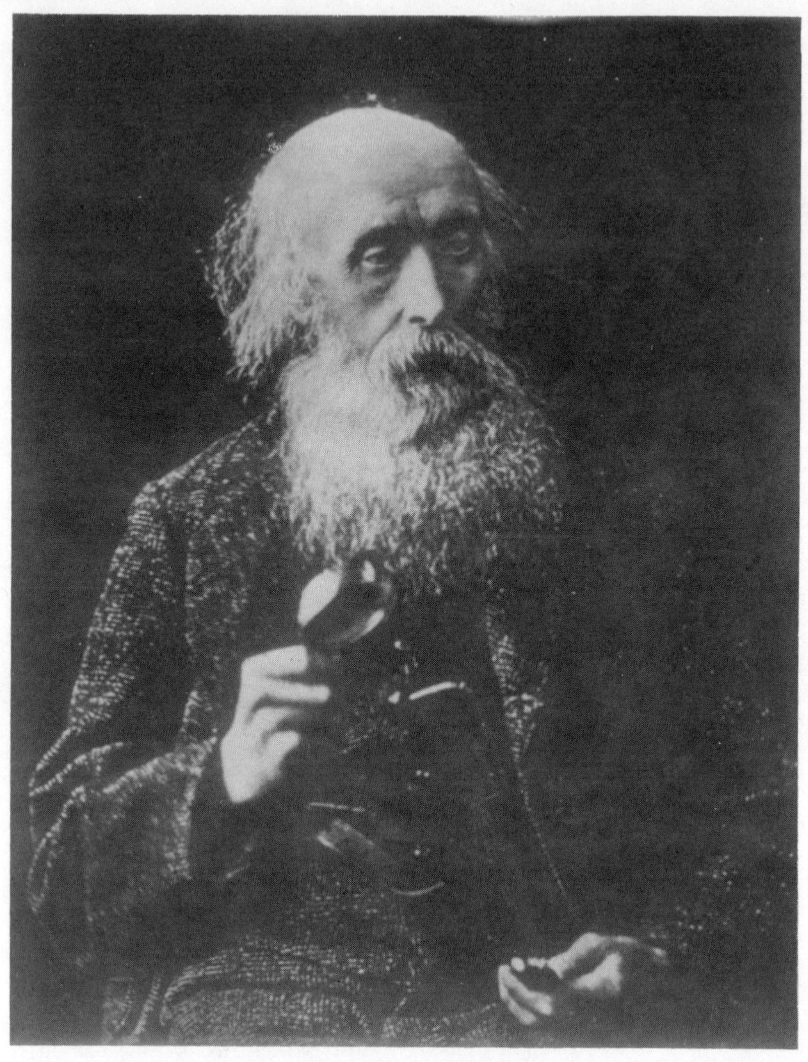

Dean John Hutton Balfour   (1808–1884)

take them when he learned that renewal of their hospital
privileges depended on their finding a medical officer willing to
assume this responsibility. He disapproved of women in medicine,
he said frankly, but he disapproved even more of the unfair way

in which the university had continuously discriminated against them after it had admitted them. And another prominent Edinburgh surgeon, too busy to take them at any other time, taught them on Sunday mornings for two winter sessions, absolutely free. Members of the die-hard opposition actually went so far as to attack this surgeon's generosity as a violation of the Sabbath, but this scheme came to nothing. Instruction of women students at the Royal Infirmary became an established practice.

It would be reasonable to assume that, with admission to the Infirmary now won, the rest would be clear sailing. But this had been only another skirmish in what was to be a very long war. Still undecided was the crucial question—would the women be allowed to graduate and receive their medical degrees?

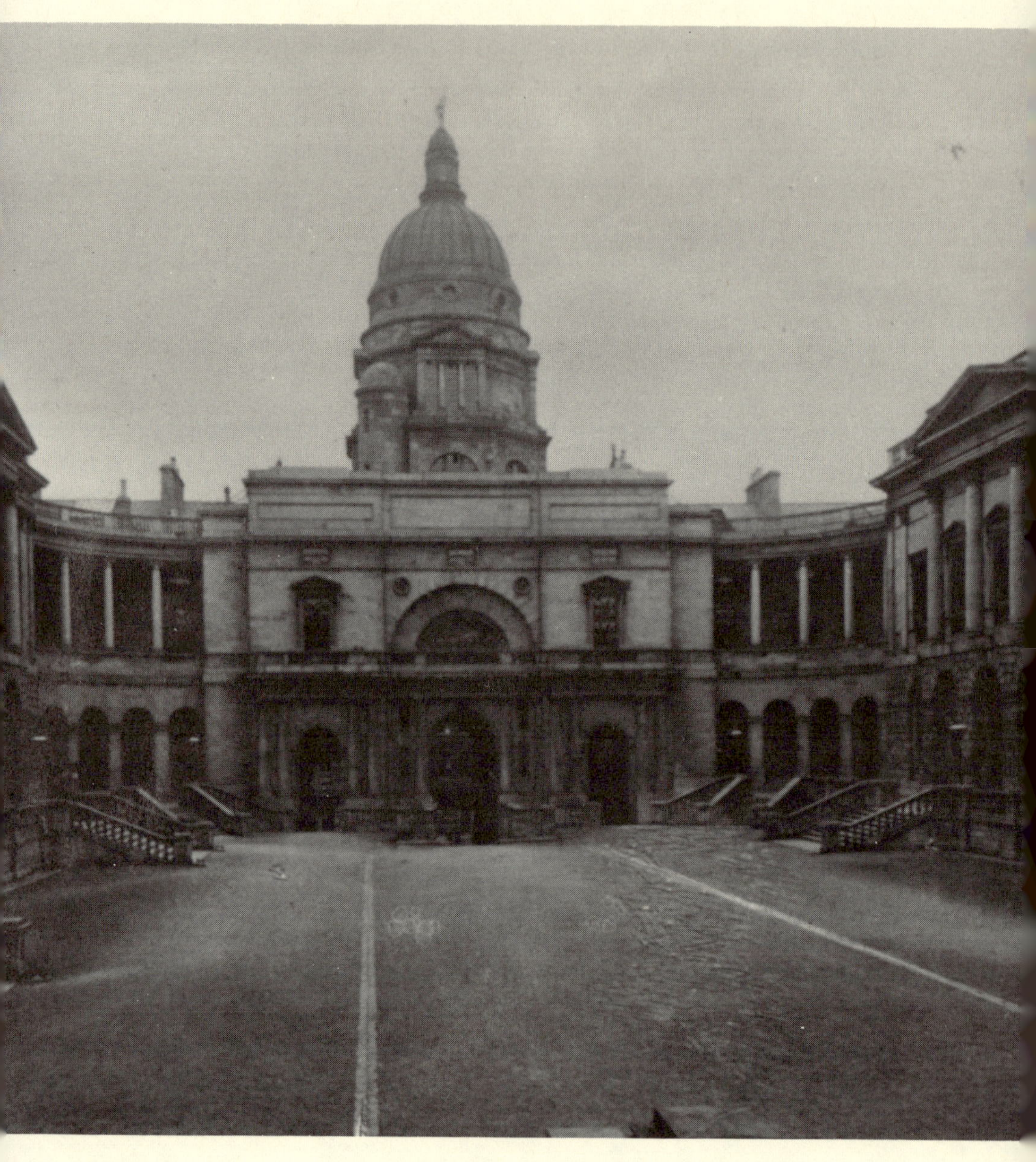

Old Quadrangle, Edinburgh University

If all the records were not so very, very clear, it would be impossible to believe that the next step taken by the university to thwart the women in their medical education was not some devilish nightmare. The women had behind them approximately two and a half years of outstanding academic performance; each barrier that had been erected along their path during those years had been overcome against enormous odds. It is a wonder that the victims of such hostility, which became more and more pronounced, did not weaken, but on the contrary became even more determined to continue their crusade. One can only guess at the toll those years of constant warfare took on the characters of those sturdy, intrepid fighters. Someone said that *iron* had entered into their souls! They continued the struggle, using every bit of talent and knowledge at their command, and solicited expert advice as needed. Each seeming victory they won was so brief—so fleeting—that before they had time to turn to the business they had come for, their education, the victory was snatched from their hands.

Even while the argument over admission was being delayed and dragged out into the spring term of 1872 by the Board of Managers of the Royal Infirmary, Sophia had made a final appeal to the University Court of Edinburgh, on behalf

6.

By Fair Means or Foul

of herself and her fellow students, to make it possible for them to complete their education. Opinion in the community had been mounting, and the lines "for" and "against" were becoming much more sharply drawn. This had the effect of increasing the reluctance of teachers to agree to lecture to the women in subjects that they still required.

And not only was there the immediate question of how the girls were to pursue their studies, but there was a larger question looming—would the women be allowed to graduate?

The University Court was unwilling to take any steps toward furthering the women's education, unless, of course, the women would agree to give up entirely the question of graduation and be content with certificates of proficiency instead of medical degrees. This the women were not ready to do, but at least they hoped to continue their studies in the meantime.

When Sophia next appealed to the University Court, she put aside the question of "ultimate graduation" and asked simply that the Court "make arrangements where we can continue our education."

With the question of graduation temporarily out of the picture, the University Court did agree to allow the women to attend separate extramural classes. Sophia tried to commit the Court to pledge that they would make every effort to see that such courses counted toward graduation "if it is subsequently determined that the University has the power of granting degrees to women," but the Court had something else in mind. The proposal of giving the women certificates of proficiency instead of allowing them to graduate and receive medical degrees had been another device to keep them from becoming doctors. Only a medical degree—and not the certificates of proficiency—would entitle the women to have their names entered in the Medical Register of the General Medical Council. Without the degree, the women would have their medical educations, but no legal right to practice medicine.

It now became abundantly clear that the medical faculty would not be budged from their position, either by public pressure or appeals to justice.

Time and again Sophia was asked whether the University "had any *right*" to put such obstructions in the women's path. Toward the end of 1871, Sophia had sought advice about bringing legal action against the University to determine once and for all whether this institution had the power to grant degrees to women. But Sophia's brother, her constant confidant, had advised against this. "You can make better use of your time," he wrote, "by getting University instruction elsewhere, than by throwing legal pebbles at the University. . . . and life being short, you had better gather up the net result of your Scotch experience, and go to Zurich or Paris . . . ."

But a degree from Zurich or Paris would not qualify the women for inclusion in the Medical Register. No, the battle must be fought here. And even Sophia's brother, once the situation had been explained to him, agreed, admitting that "there is more to be said for legal action that I knew of," but he still remained doubtful as to the possibilities of success for Sophia and her cause.

Others thought Sophia had more of a case, including the Lord Advocate of Scotland. In his opinion, a court of law would quietly "award to [Sophia and her group] what seemed unattainable by any other means."

Convinced by now that the medical faculty would do anything to get rid of them, Sophia and all the women medical students, who at this time numbered ten, initiated in March of 1872 their legal action. In legal terms, they were taking an "Action of Declarator," and so the case was known as "The Action of Declarator brought by Ten Matriculated Lady Students Against the Senatus of Edinburgh University."

When the news of this daring step became known, Sophia received a letter of protest from Dr. Elizabeth Blackwell, who urged her not to waste on an uncertain lawsuit money that might be better spent in other ways. Sophia was courteous in her reply to this woman to whom "all of us medical women owe so much gratitude and respect as our pioneer and forerunner," but she had to maintain the justness of her action, which she looked forward to explaining in detail to Dr. Blackwell.

Now a period of feverish activity began in preparation for the presentation of the case before a judge (this was not to be like an ordinary trial with witnesses and a jury; only the lawyers for each side were to appear and present their arguments, and then the judge would render his decision). Sophia was advised to search through the British Museum for any book that might give evidence of women graduates from universities. As far as Edinburgh was concerned, there was not "a single case of a woman being a student," for even though Dr. James Barry had received a medical degree there in 1812, no one had known she was a woman. Professor Nicholson, who had taught the women the extramural class in zoology, suggested that they investigate the original constitution and the official archives of the University of Bologna for "authoritative statistics on the subject" of women graduates, for this ancient Italian university, founded in the eleventh century, had been the model for Edinburgh. Sophia, with characteristic care and attention to detail, dispatched a friend on a mission to Bologna, where, Sophia told her, she was to do the following things:

1. At each University get access, if possible, to the official archives and lists of students, and make a complete list of every woman who studied there, with date, Faculty, and other particulars.

2. If you cannot get access yourself, get the lists made by some official, and, if possible, compare it with originals or other authorities.

3. If possible get the Secretary or Librarian, or some Pro-

fessor to attest the list with his signature, as truly extracted from the records.

4. Pay any necessary fees, having as far as possible arranged for these beforehand.

5. Make copies in one book of every list obtained, of name and address of each person making or attesting such lists, and of all additional information likely to be of value.

6. Send off attested lists to me in registered letters as soon as obtained, marking in your M.S. book the exact duplicate in case of loss and sending a separate letter to Miss Pechey, to announce dispatch.

7. Do not let your own M.S. book out of your hands for any purpose.

8. Send all lists on foolscap and not on foreign paper.

Sophia's ambassador seems to have carried through her mission very efficiently, for an impressive list of names was the result—more ammunition for the women's side.

On March 27 the Senatus met, soon after the lawsuit was initiated, to consider what action to take as result of the "great summons" delivered to them on behalf of the women. As Edith reported to Sophia, who was then in London, "the enemy were dreadfully angry at the lawsuit." Nonetheless, some of the Senatus members declared their sympathy with the women's cause, stating in a formal protest that they could see "no just cause for opposing the admission of women to the study and practice of medicine" and that they felt the women "should obtain what they ask—namely a complete medical education, crowned by a degree." But the majority of the Senatus was not for giving in to the women's demands and decided, instead, to oppose the women in the lawsuit.

While the lawsuit was pending back in Edinburgh, Sophia gave a lecture in London, in April of 1872, and it was here that she may have had that chance to explain her actions to Dr. Blackwell. Sophia had especially invited her to this lecture when she replied to Dr. Blackwell's protest over the lawsuit. England's other famous woman doctor, Elizabeth Garrett (now Mrs. [Dr.] Garrett Anderson), also attended. (Sophia's relationship with these two "leading ladies" of the medical profession was always somewhat precarious, and while Sophia might have wished for their enthusiastic support of all her ventures, she often, as we shall see further, had to face their opposition instead.)

"Don't have any libel cases," Edith had written to Sophia in anticipation of the lecture; "how I wish I could be in the gallery to make faces at you and throw peas!"

The chairman of this London meeting, Lord Shaftesbury, in his address, answered the argument that women were not wanted in the medical profession by saying that he was old enough to remember when railways and electric telegraphs were not wanted for the simple reason that they were not known. But when they became known and were in use, no one would think of doing without them, and "in all probability, it would be the same with reference to ladies in the medical profession!"

Perhaps Sophia had taken to heart Edith's warning about not having any libel cases, for she was on her guard this time and kept herself well under control (and was even mildly twitted for not having "worked herself up to a passion"). But the speech was a great success and was widely quoted and referred to in the newspapers.

On July 17, 1872, the lawsuit against the Senatus came before the Lord Ordinary, Lord Gifford. The lawyers for the Senatus argued that the admission of the women in the first place had been only an experiment and that the permission had been given just for partial instruction, with no view to graduation. In other words, the university existed for men only, and had never intended to allow women to be graduated. And indeed, if it had, it had had no right to. Moreover, the university really had no idea that the ten young women would insist upon *graduation*.

On July 26, 1872, nine days after the suit had begun, the judge decided in favor of the women. In handing down that decision he pointed out that "it was their demand for degrees, and their announced intention to practice medicine that had aroused unworthy jealousy and occasioned strife." The certificates of proficiency they were offered, he said, were a "mere mockery," and he hoped that, since the 1869 regulations admitting the women to the university were now declared to be in accordance with all the necessary procedures, there "would now be an end to this unfortunate controversy which had raged so long."

The women had won the lawsuit.

As always, the verdict was given much publicity, and many telegrams of congratulations once again began to come from everywhere. A Scotsman residing in India sent a thousand pounds and promised to raise more if needed, for the battle, he said, was "being gallantly fought." Sophia's brother wrote, from Switzerland, "I congratulate you heartily and hope it is final! . . . I hope your legal perils are over; and, though one has regretted that so much legal work prevented your own medical start, it has been well worth all you have gone through, or yet may go through, to open the profession thoroughly to women." He praised her "gallant stand" against what he called the "Medical Monopolists" and added: "Your . . . ability in thwarting the selfish purposes of said parties have endeared you to every liberty loving individual in the civilised world, and I sincerely hope you will long be spared to benefit suffering humanity by your experience and knowledge—knowledge which you have pursued under such tremendous difficulties but the possession of which cannot fail eventually to raise you to the very pinnacle of your profession."

The women's triumph even inspired this clever verse (with its jibes at Christison) from a poet who signed himself "A wit and a wag":

> I do rejoice, Miss Jex
> The gods have heard your Prex,
> To vindicate your Sex
> By passing a new Lex
> Though that does sadly vex
> Professor C., senex,
> Who plays the part of Rex,
> But may become an Ex,
> Because he won't annex
> The females to his Grex.

But again, as so often happened, the triumph was celebrated prematurely. The court's decision had involved the Senatus, but only the University Court had the power to establish a regulation admitting women medical students to all regular classes. This was where the legal loophole lay—the women had named only the Senatus in their lawsuit, not the entire university. Thus, as their opponents were soon to claim, the court's decision was not binding on the university as a whole.

So nothing had been settled after all. Still unresolved were the questions of whether the women would be admitted to final examinations and whether they would actually be given their degrees.

The summer of 1872 and its attendant difficulties, such as arranging classes for the next term, found Sophia left to deal with them virtually by herself. Most of the young women had scattered, some to Paris, some to Boston. Edith Pechey was working in the Lying-in Hospital in Endell Street in London. Sophia was beginning to doubt whether she herself would ever be able to finish her education. Looking ahead, she hoped that when the fight was won, she could "creep away into some wood and lie and sleep for a year." Still, she wrote, I "*must* stay at my post as long as I can stand." The hard realities of the coming months had been brought to her attention by a rather stern letter from Edith, who described her work in the hospital and then reproached

Sophia: "You have never told me how you are getting on with your exam subjects; such silence is very ominous, and I'm afraid you haven't been doing anything at them. You really must, if you intend to go up in October, for it is by no means child's play getting up three such different subjects, and it would be simply *awful* if you went up and didn't pass. . . ."

The warning was apparently not lost on Sophia, nor was she so sure of herself as she would have liked to be. She wrote to Dr. Sewall in Boston: "I am just going to get hard to work for 5 weeks in preparation for my Professional exam. which comes off about October 22nd. It would never do for *me* to be plucked! In fact I shall not go in unless I feel pretty well prepared when the time comes."

She did begin her preparation, but the time was just not opportune. The favorable decision against the university had given birth to another idea. Sophia was in the process of renting a small house to start a medical school! She was arranging for winter classes. But the new problem was to find a teacher of anatomy who would be recognized and accepted by appropriate authorities at the university, who were intent on *not* doing so. She was writing articles for newspapers, on many subjects other than the one in which she was so intimately involved. She was writing a long essay for publication, giving a detailed historical account of the entire movement among women to study and practice medicine. She was thus able to earn some money, the need for which kept growing all the time.

Early in the five weeks Sophia had allotted to preparation for her exams, she feels "rather out of heart" and "can't get courage or sense for the organic chemistry, and must leave it till E[dith] P[echey] comes; and the botany seems so desperately voluminous! My head seems tired! I *can't* make it work more than an hour or so at a time. . . . But somehow my fatalism makes me think I *shall* get through when E.P. comes and quiets me,—she comes Thursday, 10th!"

Eleven days before the dreaded exams, and this to worry about: "Such a bother about anatomy rooms, etc., and I shall have to organize about the Fund, etc. Things seem to *crowd* on me so! And other people get such nice long holidays! . . . The H. [the anatomy teacher]. The Court refused him flat on Monday, on ground of 'no evidence of qualification'! He on Tuesday is to send in his diplomas and other testimonials, and I have to get them copied and printed, etc. . . . My botany stuck fast—I was nervous and shaky again—feeling strength go out of me drop by drop! If only the 22nd [exam day] were *well* over! E. P. came back yesterday, dear child, so loving and good!"

The new women students did indifferently on their preliminary exams that October. This was a serious disappointment to Sophia, who wanted all women to shine all the time. And Sophia took the first of her exams. Then "White Millar [attorney for the women against the university] met me and worried me for law papers. Head dazed— . . . Crum Brown let me off till another day!"

The next day she took the exam in practical chemistry. Estimating her performance, she wrote, "Did good paper in Natural History, fair in chemistry; poor in botany! Went to Falkirk to sleep!"

Well, Sophia, mentally far above average in either sex, had failed in natural history, on an exam that almost any schoolboy could pass—and all eyes around the world were upon her! She found it hard to bear. She was under the impression that she had been marked unfairly. She had surely irritated some of those in authority—couldn't this be their effort to defeat her?

Thomas Henry Huxley, the English biologist, had earlier expressed sympathy for the women students, and now Edith Pechey took it upon herself to ask him for his opinion of Sophia's natural history exam paper. It was a daring gesture, and Sophia would not have permitted it had she not been confident of her performance on that examination.

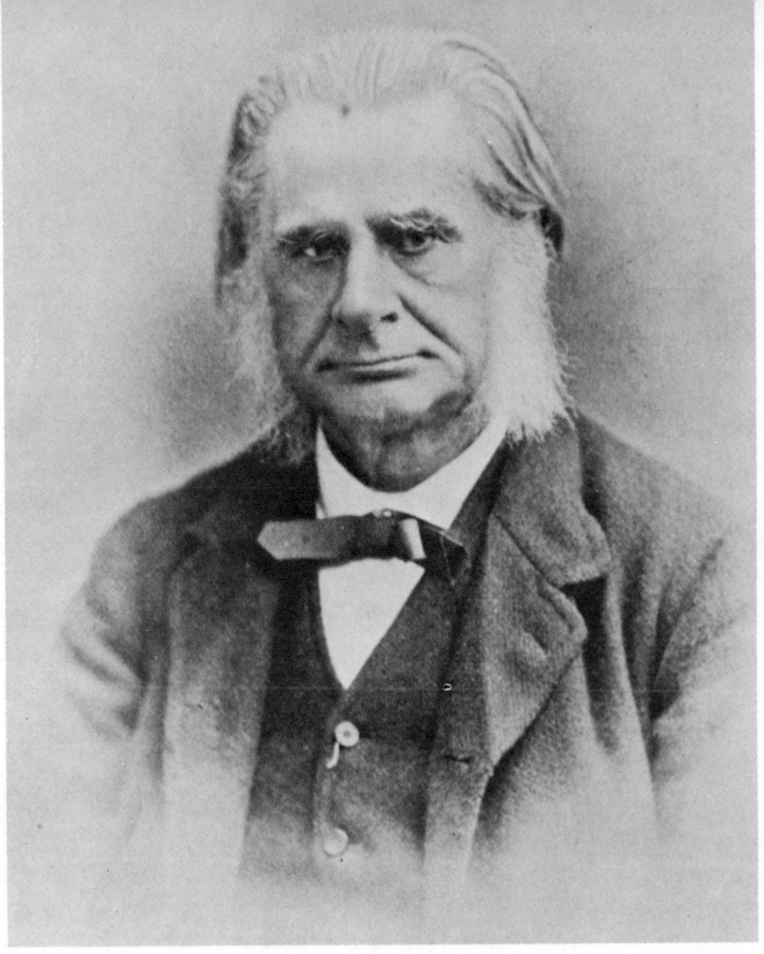

Professor Thomas Henry Huxley (1825–1895)

Edith wrote: "He said he would look over the Natural History, and although he was very kind about it, his verdict was unfavorable! Of course, I have no doubt that they would have passed a *man* on your paper, but still you must have them extra good before you can make any fuss about it. . . . I hope you won't worry yourself about the papers, as I hope we shall have plenty of leisure so that we can go over the subjects again in a proper way: it would have been a wonder if you could have passed in the midst of all that worry. . . . God bless you, darling!"

But Sophia could not reconcile herself to the way her natural history paper had been judged. She was convinced that her role in the campaign to pry open the doors of the university and bring women into the medical profession not only had cost her a passing mark but had exposed her to the ridicule of all. (The press did its utmost to spread the news, and indeed the incident was to be used later to taunt her, as we shall see.) Furthermore, the Senatus had already entered an appeal against the favorable decision previously rendered to the women by the law court. Now, more certain than ever that the university had resolved to get rid of them, by fair means or foul, Sophia and a friend went on a scouting trip to other universities in Scotland to urge for admission.

Edith returned to Edinburgh to find Sophia away on her mission to St. Andrews University and Newcastle. So, with the university's appeal about to take place, Edith informed Sophia that "last night Millar sent a copy of the Lords' Opinion with a note to say that the case would be put on this week, and that the proceedings would occupy only a few minutes—merely formal. He is to let me know when it comes on. Ormidale, Mure, Mackenzie and Shand [very likely the same Shand who had been Craig's counsel in the libel suit] are dead against us, contending that the Court had no power to make the regulations. Deas, Armillan, Jerviswoode and Gifford only in favor of the regulations holding good and our right to graduation—but *not* a word as to the regulations being enforced, and we are still left at the mercy of the individual professors."

Meanwhile, Sophia, not surprisingly, had received absolute refusals from the universities outside of Edinburgh. The women were even urged to get their classes somehow, anyhow, and then to "practice boldly as unregistered practitioners who are ready to submit to examination when called upon." Mrs. Thorne was doing her best to get classes going at Edinburgh and, in case degrees proved to be out of the question, was investigating whether the women might obtain the license of the Royal Colleges of Physicians and Surgeons, a privilege which was not granted until some dozen years later. The women were reaching out in all possible directions that year. Not a stone was left unturned. The women's diligence coupled with much restraint was admirable.

In October of 1873 Edith wrote to Sophia from her home in Langham, now giving vent to her feelings: "Since I saw you, I have indeed suffered many things of many physicians, and my temper is no better but rather worse. It is, however, gradually working down to its normal again. If I could only have spoken my mind when they talked their conceited bosh about their infinite superiority, and said—'Do you know what a poor fool you are making of yourself?' It wouldn't have been so hard; but to sit still, smiling benignantly, when men, commonplace enough, goodness knows, in everything but their uncommon stupidity boasted of their mental capacity! . . . Still I would not have Mrs. Thorne stop in her arrangements for classes in Edinburgh, as I think we have no chance, the influence of the medical men being so much against us."

The great decision on the university's appeal was finally given. Seven of the twelve judges voted in favor of the Senatus, and the women lost. The previous ruling that had judged the university regulations admitting women as having been properly adopted was now reversed. According to this new decision, the university had *not* had the right to formulate such rules, and therefore these women should not have been admitted to the university. Not only did the women lose the case, they also lost their places at the university, and, in addition, they were ordered to pay the court costs of £848 6s. 8d.!

And so ended the hard-fought battle of Edinburgh.

The scene now switches to London.

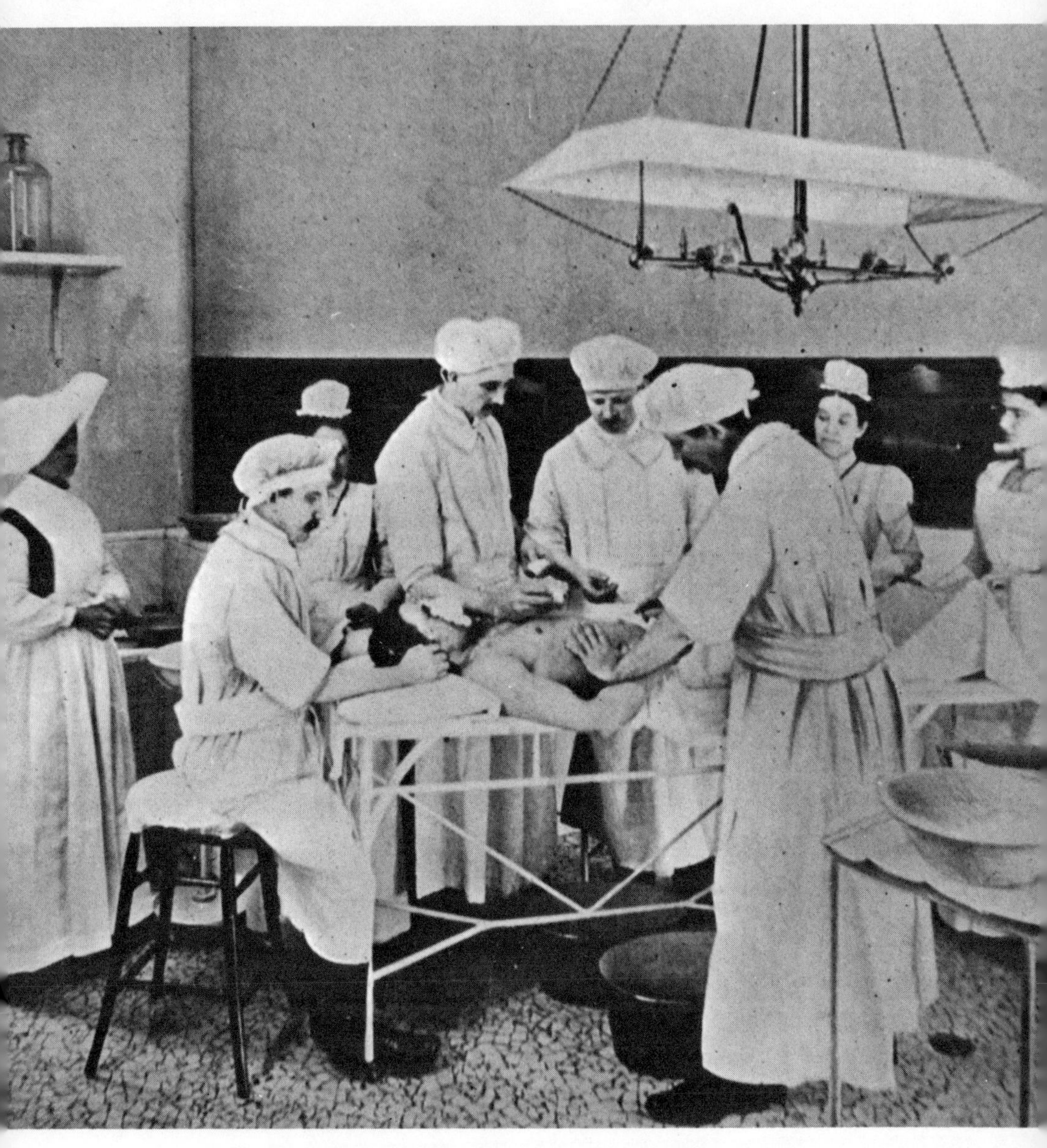

Gaining admittance to a recognized hospital for clinical training was one of the many hurdles the pioneering women had to challenge.

When the University of Edinburgh had made crystal clear its intention to get rid of the women at all costs (the reversal of the law court's verdict having given the administration the basis for doing so) and Sophia had been rebuffed in her search through universities with medical schools in Scotland, she then turned to the eleven medical schools in London. By this time we all know the outcome—a sharp refusal! However, in that process, here and there she found individual professors who wanted to help her and actually did so, to their everlasting credit.

Dr. T. King Chambers of St. Mary's Hospital in Scotland had known of her efforts to get a medical education since the very beginning in 1869, when he was attending her mother in that lady's most continuous illnesses. At that time he had made inquiries on Sophia's behalf about admission to the medical school of St. Mary's but had been bluntly refused. Now in 1874 she turned to him again for help in her new project—founding a medical school for women in London. He introduced her to Dr. A. T. Norton. Their meeting was one of the most decisive steps in that new undertaking. Norton was a doctor; he was called "Dr." Norton because in Britain the title of "Mr." is reserved for surgeons only. Norton had associated himself with the work at Elizabeth Garrett Anderson's hospital since its

7.

London and Ireland

inception. He was a consultant there and knew that women could—and should—play an important part in medical practice.

Mr. (Dr.) Anstie, another supporter, had for some time been encouraging Sophia to undertake such a step, suggesting that she try to raise enough money from friends and sympathizers, in which event, if she succeeded, he himself—and he was sure that there would be others—would be willing to teach at the school. It was a gamble, but he thought that this would convince all friends, as well as opponents, of the earnestness and sincerity of the women and that eventually some hospitals would be willing to admit them for clinical training.

In the early months of 1874 some people argued that Sophia was unwise in embarking on the ambitious project of founding a medical school for women in London when two of England's most respected women doctors, Elizabeth Garrett Anderson and Elizabeth Blackwell, were opposed to doing so at that time. These two doctors, who had already achieved so much, tended to view the women's struggle in more personal terms and were out of sympathy with Sophia's grand plans to win admission to the medical profession not only for herself, but, as she put it, "for all!" Mrs. Thorne, on her return from Paris, where she had been spending the summer of 1874, also tried to dissuade Sophia. But once Sophia got her teeth into something, she was not easily persuaded to let go. An organizational meeting was held in Mr. Anstie's house on August 22, 1874. Mrs. Thorne came, and so did Edith Pechey, and also Norton and King Chambers, among others. A provisional committee was set up, and it was unanimously resolved that it was "desirable that a school be founded in London with a view to educating women in medicine and enabling them to pass such examinations as would place their names on the Medical Register." The plan was to open the school on October 12, 1874—less than two months away.

Sophia realized that Mrs. (Dr.) Garrett Anderson (who the previous year had become the first woman elected to membership in the British Medical Association) and Elizabeth Blackwell would somehow have to be induced to lend their names to the provisional committee. She wrote them that for their own reputations as well as for the proposed school it would be advisable to present a united front. (Then she added that the school would be set up whether or not they agreed to serve on the committee.) They were faced with no alternative but to agree, but they stated conditions that, in effect, deprived Sophia of any official position other than that of trustee. They insisted that registered practitioners only should constitute the provisional committee. From previous experience in dealing with Sophia, they had grave misgivings about working closely with her.

Contemporary critics of Sophia's "difficult character," of her unwillingness to accept lasting defeat in anything she undertook, often found her stubbornness irritating. These same critics would admit that she encouraged them to be truthful when she asked for advice about her future plans, but, said they, it was almost impossible to differ with her or to suggest alternatives. She did not take kindly to adverse criticism, and furthermore generally found ways to argue people out of opposing positions. Sophia was called obstinate, irritating, stubborn, difficult, unwilling to listen to what her critics called "reason"—but perhaps this has been true of many great thinkers of the past who have succeeded in moving mankind's thinking forward, sometimes against its own will.

And so, in the beginning at least, Sophia's name was not to be publicly or officially connected with the proposed medical school. Plans for the school would have to be submitted to the provisional committee, on which she had no vote; nonetheless, Sophia undertook to do all the secretarial work that was involved.

Sophia and Mrs. Thorne already had persuaded fourteen friends to contribute £100 each (about $500, at that time), and this was the capital with which the project was started. A staff had also been recruited and was willing to teach. Twelve students who had been at Edinburgh and several others were waiting for admission. But when the organizational meeting was held on August 22, a building had not yet been found.

Less than four weeks later, however, on September 15, after tramping from one agent to another with her unceasing energy and determination, Sophia signed a lease and took possession of a building at 30 Henrietta Street, a quiet little street at that time, far enough away from noisy thoroughfares. The building, which had the added advantage of being within easy reach of museums and libraries, stood in the middle of a large garden and had a verandah running the length of the ground floor. Legend has it that King George IV had used the house as the residence of his mistresses. Sophia's diary records that, after signing the lease, she rigged up a bed "and slept there that night." Early in October Sophia moved into a house at 32 Bernard Street that she had taken as her private residence.

Between September 15, when Sophia found the building on Henrietta Street, and October 12, when the school was to open, much would have to be done. Alterations had to be made, and Sophia supervised them all. She knew about plumbing and was enough of a technician in other house-building matters to know how much to expect from the workmen and to demand that they do it. And they did! Sophia recorded the feat in these simple words: "October 12th, Monday, Opening of the London School of Medicine for Women."

On October 12, fourteen students just walked in and began their work. There was no formal opening and not even an inaugural lecture. One wonders whether this lack of ceremony was in deference to the death of Mr. Anstie, which had come with tragic suddenness only three days before Sophia had signed the lease on the house. His loss could have proved fatal, but A. T. Norton stepped into the breach, accepted the post of dean, and worked hard for the success of the school's objectives. Some years later, an entry in the minutes of the School Council, the London School's governing body, recorded, speaking in retrospect of Norton's having taken the post as dean: "[For him] to do so at that time, when prejudice against the movement was strong and active, required much courage and determination." These qualities, plus his natural tact and good judgment, no doubt served him well in the difficult early years of that tremendous undertaking.

In the very first session, the winter of 1874–1875, nine additional students enrolled, bringing the student body to twenty-three. The plan of study had been worked out by the lecturers, who were, fortunately, men of unusual ability already teaching in recognized schools. The required subjects would be covered in three years, and the curriculum included four subjects more than the examining boards required.

Even with the greatest economy possible and generous help from sympathetic supporters, the project was often in great danger. One reason was that fees to lecturers were guaranteed, a most unusual procedure. Furthermore, additional reconstruction of the school building was required. The income from the students' fees was insufficient, and more money had to be sought from friends in Edinburgh and London. In fact, the students themselves were so hard-pressed for money that, after much discussion, the school itself granted them £10 apiece for the purchase of books.

No doubt, lack of funds troubled the provisional committee. But lack of money was not the most serious problem. The survival of the school actually depended upon two even more important requirements. The first was finding an examining body among the nineteen that would agree to allow the women to take their examinations. And this meant, in effect, recognition that the school was providing the proper standard of medical education. Secondly, a hospital had to be found that would be willing to admit the women to clinical training. And this, too, meant acknowledging that the school was meeting the academic requirements for medical education.

As soon as the school opened, the dean wrote to each of the nineteen examining boards in London and asked that the school be placed on their list of accredited and recognized medical schools. All nineteen refused.

If the school was meeting with rebuffs on the one hand, it was also gaining the support of some noted people, on the other. One of these was James B. Stansfeld of the Liberal Party, Member of Parliament for Halifax. Sophia had first met him in the days preceding the Edinburgh libel trial. Later, as we shall see, his help and his influence were to prove priceless.

In May of 1875 the provisional committee was changed to a permanent council, and men and women prominent in world affairs and in Parliament who favored the women's cause were added to its membership. Among these was Lord Shaftesbury, one of the most outstanding liberals of the time, who had presided at the 1872 London meeting where Sophia had lectured. His enthusiastic support of the school was especially noticed by the public on June 2, 1875, when he distributed prizes that some of the women students had earned during the school's first session in the winter of 1874–1875. (Sophia must have felt this was a welcome change from the atmosphere at Edinburgh, where leading members of the faculty had twice refused to appear at such ceremonies if the women were to be present to receive their prizes.) Shaftesbury reminded his audience of the great difficulties the courageous women had overcome, which, he said, their characters as well as the medical profession would be all the better for having gone through.

But there were many problems still to be overcome. A relatively minor one concerned the landlord of the school building, who had heard gossip that one of the rooms was used for dissection, a practice that was not looked upon with favor in those days, even by some sections of the profession. He would have

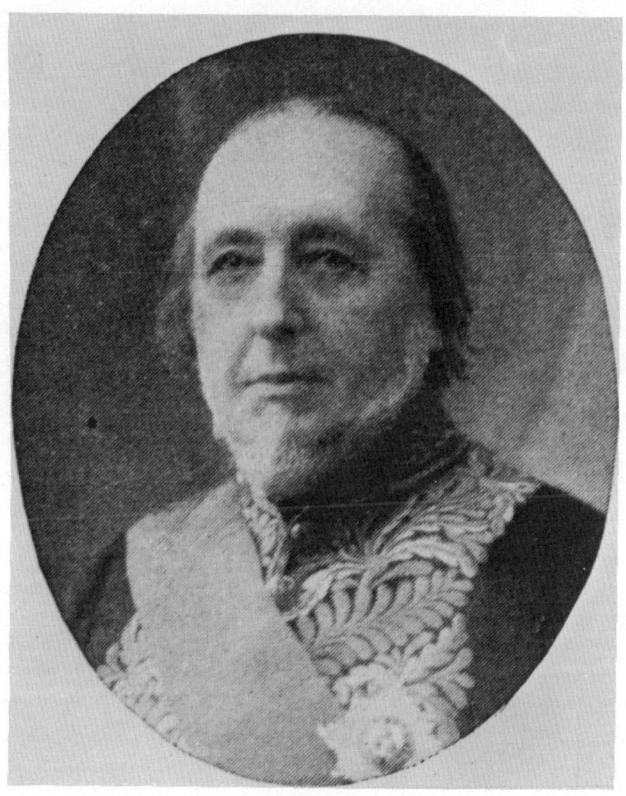

Sir James Stansfeld   (1820–1898)

to be appeased without jeopardizing the school's right to continue with dissection.

But the largest problems of all—greater than the need for funds or anything else—were those of gaining admission to the examinations given by the nineteen authorized boards and gaining admission to hospitals for clinical training. One of the resourceful members of the school's council had a plan. He learned that, according to present law, the midwifery license encompassed the same curriculum as that at regular medical schools, offered the same qualification as a license in medicine, and entitled those who held it to have their names in the Medical Register and to practice legally as doctors. He urged Sophia, Edith, and Mrs.

Thorne, who had completed the medical courses in Edinburgh over a period of almost four years and who had received a set of certificates of attendance for each of the courses, to apply for admission to the College of Surgeons for its license in midwifery. The women were agreed that such a license by itself was not a desirable or dignified way of entering the profession, but it seemed to be the only way open at the moment, and not to take advantage of that possibility would be a mistake. Furthermore, it could mean a lot to the London School. The more women who could be licensed, the greater would be the growth of the school, until, finally, reason would hopefully prevail among the nineteen examining bodies and the hostile doctors.

Once again Sophia led the way, being the first to apply to take the examination for the midwifery license. She, Edith, and Mrs. Thorne began to brush up on their midwifery studies, while the College of Surgeons consulted legal authorities. When the answer came, it was, at last, good news. The women could take the examination and be granted certificates as licentiates in midwifery, and this would entitle them to be included in the Medical Register. Success was within sight. Sophia's diary on Friday, January 21, 1876, tells us that it is her thirty-sixth birthday and that "it seems as if this year was really to gain . . . what I have been fighting for in England for 7 years—Registration!"

It did indeed look as though victory was around the corner. The women's applications to take the examination were accepted. It seemed as though the way was clear. And then—*the whole board of examiners resigned.* No examinations were scheduled. No one would agree to serve on a new board of examiners. Even a year later (1877) there were no examiners to be found, and there was no examination. And no licensing examination was scheduled—or given—during the next ten years.

The College of Surgeons had seemed the ideal "back door" to inclusion in the Medical Register—but that door had just slammed shut. Edith Pechey, who then held a post at the

Women's Hospital in Birmingham under Mr. Lawson Tait, wrote, "Perhaps after all it is as well, as . . . that [license] would have been a sorry thing to practice upon. . . ."

Luckily, too, all was not lost, for the women had earlier made some inquiries on what was to be a promising new front—Ireland.

And also some new figures appeared on the Irish scene during these troubled years when the London School was just beginning. In January of 1874 Louisa Atkins had requested the King's and Queen's College of Physicians of Ireland to recognize the diploma of the University of Zurich, a foreign university, as qualification for admission to the final examination for the license in midwifery. After much argument back and forth, and the by now customary passing and subsequent rescinding of motions, it was finally agreed that Miss Atkins might take the examination for a license in midwifery. On August 6, 1874, another woman presented herself: "Miss Mary Ellen Greenstreet was examined orally by examiners—after which they consulted and certified that [she] should be allowed the License to practice as Midwife and Nurse-tender."

On November 6, 1874, Mr. Norton, Dean of the London School of Medicine for Women, asked that his school be posted on the list of medical schools recognized by King's and Queen's College. The Irish college replied that his request was premature, since they had "not resolved to admit women as candidates for the License in Medicine."

Licensing in medicine was to be another major issue, and, in fact, the college would soon be taken to task for having even granted Miss Greenstreet her license in midwifery. Progress, as usual, was slow on the academic front, and while Edith Pechey was negotiating with the Irish college, an act of Parliament was passed that permitted universities and medical schools to admit women, if they chose to do so; the decision was left to each individual university and medical school. Edith petitioned the

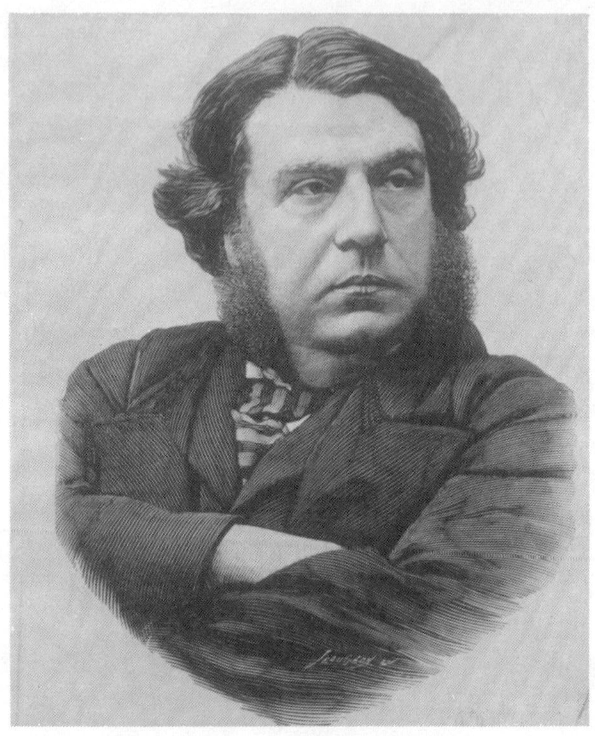

Robert Lawson Tait   (1845–1899)

college in the fall of 1876 "to avail themselves of the new power" granted by this act and to admit her to the examination for the license in medicine. And they granted her this permission! While she was waiting for the scheduling of the examination for this license, the London School of Medicine for Women petitioned the college to recognize its lectures "when presented by Female candidates for the License of the College." Things were moving fast now, thanks to the new act of Parliament, and as the young women who had studied at Edinburgh moved closer to registration, the London School was making parallel progress.

On December 1, 1876, the Inspection Committee of King's and Queen's College recommended that permission be granted to Elizabeth Walker Dunbar, M.D., Zurich, 1872, to be examined for the license of the college. The motion was carried by the deciding vote of the college president. Here at last was the first real victory! Elizabeth Walker Dunbar of Clifton, Bristol, England, even with her University of Zurich degree of 1872, was, on January 10, 1877, *the very first woman in Great Britain admitted to the Irish license in medicine.*

At that same meeting, the college agreed that a "personal inspection" of the London School of Medicine for Women and "its appliances for teaching" would have to be carried out before it could consider a decision on admitting its students to the licensing examinations.

The women's progress in this period seems to have taken place in monthly jumps as the college held each of its many meetings. The next step was to occur at the February 2, 1877, meeting, where Frances Elizabeth Hoggan, M.D., Zurich, 1870, and Louisa Atkins, Zurich, 1872, were given permission to take examinations for the *license to practice medicine,* "the College considering their qualifications in midwifery sufficient to satisfy the By Laws." Now that was victory for the second and third women, at long, long last! At that meeting Dr. A. Smith made a report of his personal inspection of the London School of Medicine for Women and stated his opinion that the details of teaching and appliances were satisfactory. A motion that the college accept certificates of lectures delivered at that school was then made and passed.

While the King's and Queen's College of Physicians was holding meetings, Edith and Sophia, in the winter of 1876, had finally gone to the University of Bern to take examinations there for the M.D. degree—which they had to take in German! Now Edith presented the Irish college with a Bern degree and asked to be admitted to the final examination in midwifery.

Zurich had been recognized by the Irish college, but Bern was another matter. And so more meetings were held, during which the women's opponents took the familiar action of trying to have earlier decisions in favor of the women rescinded.

Finally, Bern was added to the list of acceptable foreign universities (along with Geneva), and as a holder of an M.D. degree, Edith could take the examination for the license of the college. Edith Pechey's application and her papers were found to be in accordance with the bylaws, and she would be "admitted to the final examination for the Licence on presenting the certificate of practical midwifery." The chronic amenders tried once again to postpone consideration of her application for six months, but failed. On May 9, 1877, she was examined orally, "after which the Censors consulted and certified that Miss Pechey should be allowed the Licence to practice Medicine." And with her on that very day, Sophia Jex-Blake was licensed. On May 10 at 4 P.M. Edith was examined orally in midwifery, and she passed. The King's and Queen's College of Physicians' Roll of Licentiates in Medicine shows, after the names of Elizabeth Dunbar and Frances Hoggan: No. 1830—Louisa Atkins, the third woman, on May 9, 1877; No. 1831—Mary Edith Pechey, of Langham, Colchester, the fourth woman, same date; and No. 1832—Sophia Jex-Blake of London, the fifth woman, on that same date!

Without further delay—at long last—the London School of Medicine for Women was placed on the college's list of recognized medical schools, and let it be said to the everlasting credit of King's and Queen's College of Physicians (now the Irish College of Physicians) that despite repeated attempts to delay and even thwart the process, it was the very first college in Great Britain to accord that school in London the crucial help so vital to its growth and survival. It was also the first college in Great Britain to admit women with foreign university degrees to its examinations and grant them licenses to practice medicine. So at last the problem of licensing was solved, but hospital training for the London School still had to be arranged.

In the early weeks of the school's existence, application had been made to the London Hospital, which had more beds than the male medical students needed. The request was that certain wards be set aside to train the women. Even the intervention of Mrs. Garrett Anderson did not overcome the opposition of the conservative medical staff, and the application was rejected.

Next to the school, on Gray's Inn Road, was the Royal Free Hospital, and it was the next one to be approached; but the medical staff declined even "to entertain the question." Of course, Mrs. Garrett Anderson's New Hospital for Women would have been glad to admit the women, but it did not have even the minimum number of beds that the law required for clinical training of doctors.

James Stansfeld, then treasurer of the London School (in addition to being a member of Parliament), came to the rescue at this point. As luck would have it, while on a holiday he met the chairman of the Royal Free Hospital's board, who was also on a holiday, with his wife. The chairman had known nothing about the medical staff's summary dismissal of the school's request and promised to call a meeting to consider the women's application. On March 10, 1877, Stansfeld sent a telegram to Sophia: ROYAL FREE HOSPITAL HAVE UNANIMOUSLY ACCEPTED MY PROPOSAL. It was a wonderful victory! The hospital had driven a hard bargain, though, and the London School had had to agree to some demanding financial terms, but the removal of that last barrier to the school's survival was worth it. Now all that was needed were earnest, hard-working, serious women who intended to practice medicine.

In contrast to the rather simple opening of the school in October of 1874, now, in October, 1877, there was indeed an inaugural address—a brilliant speech delivered by Dr. Edith Pechey. Recalling the male students she and her group had known all too well at Edinburgh, she said she took it for granted "that there are no unwilling daughters driven here much against the grain by the commands of inexorable fathers . . . and who must

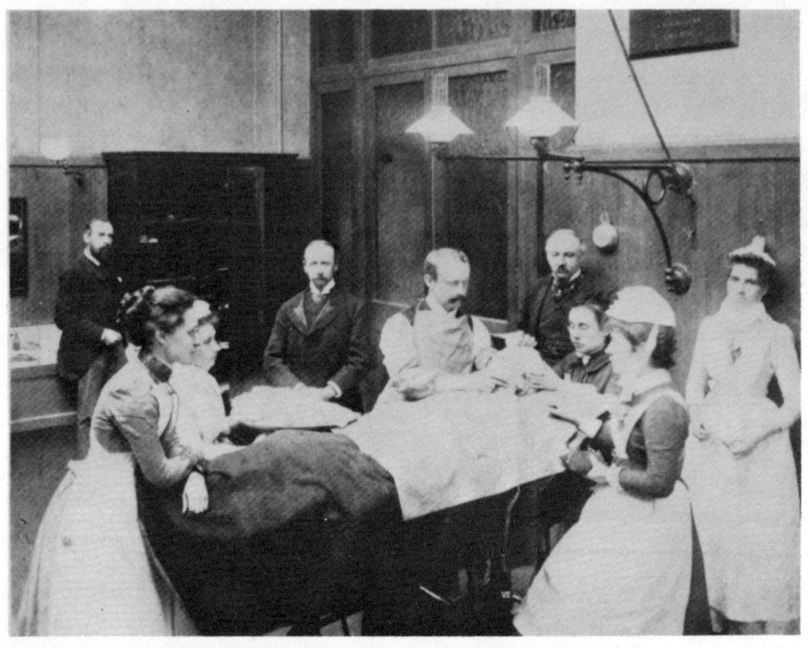

The London School of Medicine for Women: clinical instruction as it was given in the late 1800s.

be warned against the distractions of beer and billiards! . . ." She emphasized her hope that the young students would expand their knowledge of all the sciences, saying she would "rather believe that you are all animated with the desire of leaving the world better and richer and wiser for your presence in it . . . ," and she urged them to dedicate themselves "to do what in you lies, in however and humble and small a way, to further the prevention and cure of disease!"

The London School of Medicine for Women experienced a steady growth from the time it was founded by our brave, stalwart handful of women, led by Sophia Jex-Blake, and the important people she had succeeded in winning over to her crusade. Despite the expense of financing a medical education for women over the long period of, at first, three years and then four (exclusive of the clinical training of at least one year), enrollment in the school increased with every new session. By 1887—thirteen years after the school had opened with 14 students—there were 77 young women enrolled. Two years later there were 91; three years later there were 133; in 1896, an unprecedented entry of 50 new students brought the total student body to 159. In 1903 there were 318 students, and in 1917 the number had grown to 441! By any yardstick this was tremendous success.

Not only had the women won the right to a medical education, to hospital training, and to inclusion in the Medical Register, but they had also brought the entire subject of education to the fore; they had involved Parliament itself in the question. The women had some highly placed friends, some outstanding members of Parliament, on their side, but as we shall see, Parliament was soon to threaten to take away with one bill what they had granted to the women with another. Let us take a look inside the Houses of Parliament and see how the women's cause was faring.

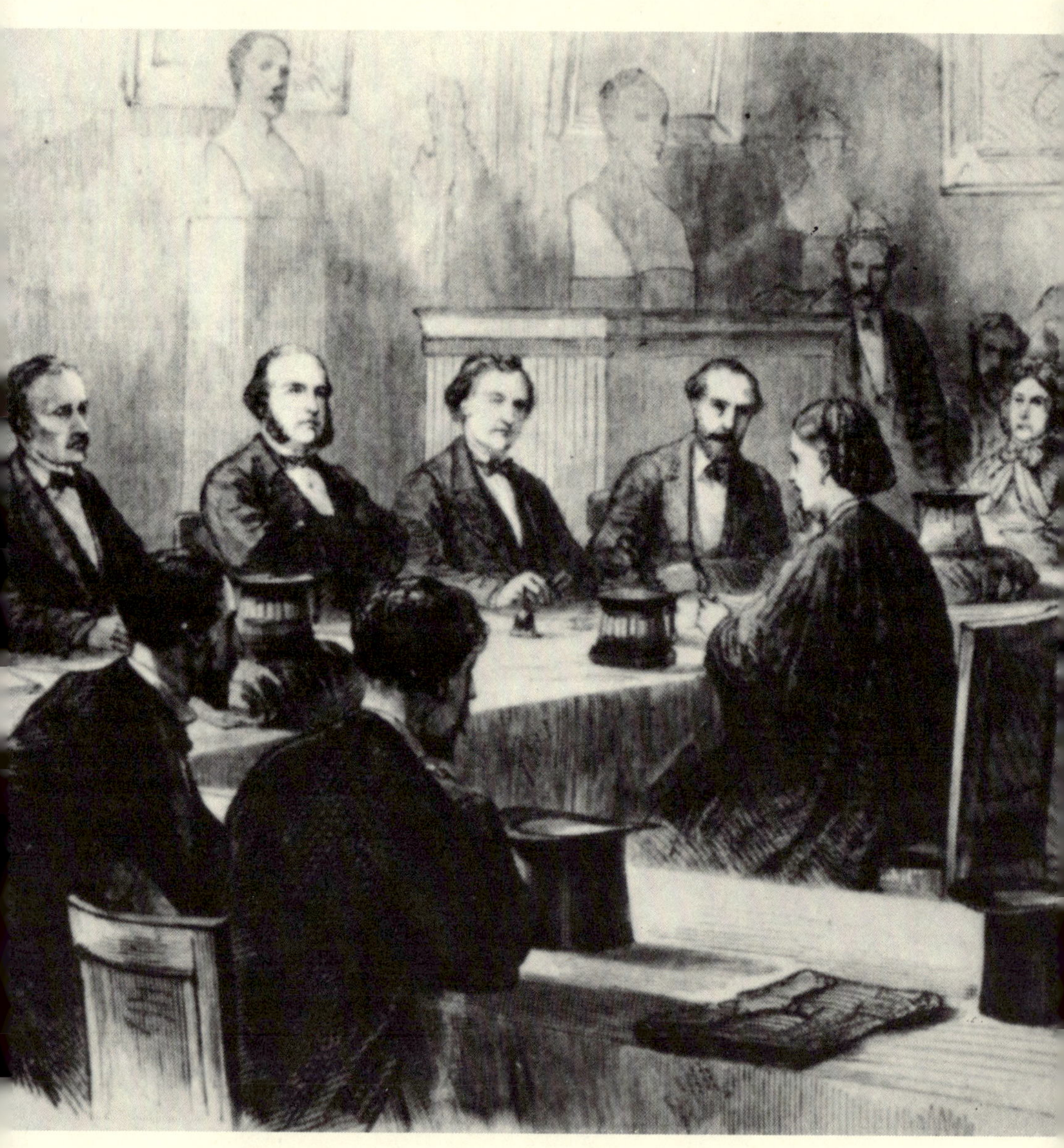

Elizabeth Garrett taking her oral examinations for her M.D. in Paris, June 1870

The women had won their important victories for the London School of Medicine for Women by the end of March, 1877, and to some extent Parliament had been involved in creating an atmosphere more favorable to their cause; Parliament had first become actively involved in 1872, when Sophia, Edith, and the other women were still in Edinburgh.

In August, 1872, during a debate in the House of Commons on appropriations, Sir David Wedderburn, who was friendly to the women medical students' cause, proposed that the funds of the University of Edinburgh should be reduced by the amount of the salaries of the medical professors, because of their inexcusable conduct. Though he dropped this proposal when it appeared that the court verdict in favor of the women would smooth the way for them at Edinburgh, that city's university, as we know, appealed the verdict and won a reversal. So Wedderburn announced that at the next session of Parliament he would introduce a bill to grant the Scottish universities the power they were now supposed not to have, namely, that of giving women a medical education and granting them regular medical degrees.

With the shift of scene from Edinburgh to Parliament, the cause was plunged into practical politics, which had the effect of inducing newspapers

8.

The Women Appeal to Parliament

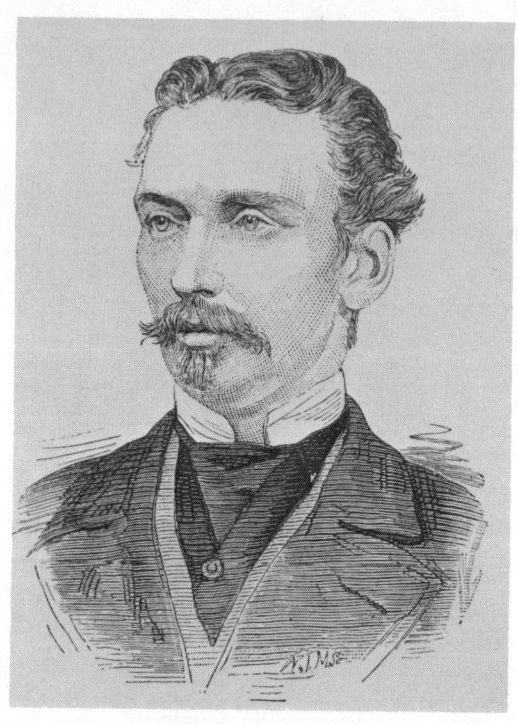

Sir David Wedderburn   (1835–1882)

and medical journals to publish articles and take sides either for or against the women, and so did members of Parliament.

Sophia realized the importance of obtaining Government support for any bill that might be introduced to promote her cause. She began to gain such support by writing to the Home Secretary in London. He agreed to do what he could to forward her views, even to the extent of introducing an appropriate bill, though he admitted his constituents might find it "not . . . very agreeable." James Stansfeld, the man who had helped the London School gain admission to the Royal Free Hospital and who had been a longtime supporter of the women's cause, advised Sophia to come to London to interview members of the Government before the January, 1873, cabinet meetings.

In the midst of her conferences with various individuals in government, Sophia's presence in Brighton was required at the bedside of her mother, who was suddenly taken very ill. Happily, her mother recovered, and in the meantime the work in London went on quietly.

During her stay in London, Sophia had been consulting with lawyers for their help in drafting a suitable bill. By April of 1874 it was ready, and Sophia's influence is reflected in its title: "A Bill to Remove Doubts as to the Powers of the Universities of Scotland to Admit Women as Students, and to Grant Degrees to Women." The bill was technically known as an "enabling bill," that is, one that would *enable* universities to admit women rather than *compel* them to do so. It was introduced into the House of Commons by another staunch defender of the women's cause—W. Cowper-Temple, who had taken a leading part in formulating the Medical Reform Act of 1858, and of whom we shall hear more later. Supporters in Parliament hoped the bill would slip through quietly, even though that seemed unlikely, too much to count on. When the bill was introduced into Parliament, news of it flashed throughout Scotland. Sixty-five petitions in favor of the bill were handed to Parliament almost immediately. One petition in favor was signed by twenty-six professors from Scottish universities, half of them from the University of Edinburgh itself. Four petitions were received that were against the bill—from the University Court, from the Senatus, and from the medical faculty of the University of Edinburgh, and also one from the University of Glasgow.

Sir Robert Christison, speaking during the debate in Parliament, called the bill a misrepresentation: "There are no such doubts," he said. The University Court, he declared, "has decided that the admission of women to study or graduate is contrary to their charters"—and this decision, we might recall, was largely a result of his own opposition to the women students.

Despite the fact that the opposing petitions were far out-

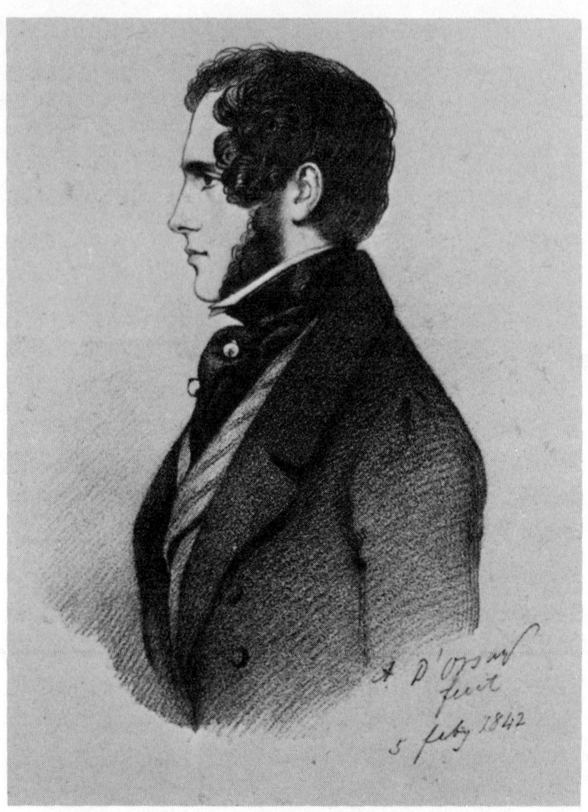

W. Cowper-Temple   *(1811–1888)*

numbered, the opponents of the bill had a clever leader in the Member of Parliament for the University of Edinburgh, Dr. Lyon Playfair, and he managed, temporarily at least, to turn the tide in the opponents' favor. All bills must be read three times in Parliament before debate, discussion, and voting can take place. By slyly maneuvering to get a postponement of the second reading of the bill (in the face of a crowded parliamentary calendar), Playfair managed to make action on the bill impossible in the current session, and so almost an entire year was lost.

On March 3, 1875, the enabling bill was again brought into Parliament. A long debate followed. Every cliché—weaker sex, smaller brain, modesty and delicacy of feeling, sure to be violated by the practice of medicine, women's "place in nature to which the Almighty in His omnipotent wisdom had called them"—echoed and reechoed solemnly. There were statements motivated by prejudice, and some, such as this one, motivated by noble sentiments: A member named Arthur Roebuck addressed his colleagues, saying, "We are here a body of men deciding upon the interests of the community, and we ought not forget that in spite of ourselves, the feeling of our own sex rises up, and men's interest are preferred to women's . . . in spite of all the soothing words we hear; and men will desire to do that for men which they will not do for women. You may talk for a month; you may bring great law to bear upon this question; you may quote names great in history, arts and science. But you cannot rub out the stain which will be on this House if it refuses to do justice to women . . . and prevents them [from] using [their] intellect . . . in a fair, honest, and upright manner for their own good."

Another member of Parliament was convinced that he was stating on good authority that "women are fitted by Nature and by God to be nurses! Let them remain so! God sent women to be ministering angels, to soothe the pillow, minister the palliative, whisper words of comfort to the tossing patient ill with fever. Let that continue to be woman's work. Leave the physician's function, the scientific lore, the iron wrist and iron will to men!" Therefore, the argument continued, there was no need to change whatever the University of Edinburgh was doing. And furthermore, no changes should be made in the universities of Scotland that were not at the same time made in all the universities of the United Kingdom!

It was suggested, rather logically, during the debate that the matter could be approached more intelligently if the members took account of certain facts: namely, that the number of physicians had been declining steadily over the past few years and that at the same time the death rate was growing steadily higher. This situation raised a valid question—if there were not enough male candidates for the physician's license, why then refuse women candidates who were eager to practice medicine? They had certainly demonstrated their ability to achieve academically at least the same high level as men and, more often, even higher levels, for which the honor lists of the University of Edinburgh provided irrefutable evidence.

Another member stated that "the duty of prescribing and dictating medical treatment had, by instinct and commonsense, fallen to men! Was it not better to be a nurse like Florence Nightingale than . . . one of those she-doctors, elbowing her way in the world with masculine activity?"

Lyon Playfair, the wily member for the University of Edinburgh, let the cat out of the bag when he raised this highly charged point: "If [the enabling bill] became law tomorrow, it would be useless in the attainment of its purpose. . . . What is the use of conferring powers upon [universities] which they do not want, and which they could not exercise if they possessed them?"

James Stansfeld in his remarks argued that the question involved two distinct aspects; the first was one of public policy. In other words, university education for women was a matter for consideration by Parliament. The local authorities, however, should work out the best way of accomplishing this policy. He added that women were not prevented by law from carrying on any business. So Parliament should avoid artificial restrictions that would deny them the right to enter professions of their choice.

The second aspect was one involving the private grievances of the women students. Women, he said, should be permitted to train to become doctors, and Parliament should create the conditions to enable them to do so. There was no doubt that male doctors were jealous of women who aspired to become qualified physicians. And the grievances the women held against the University of Edinburgh were justified because the university had not played fair with them. After having used every legal means

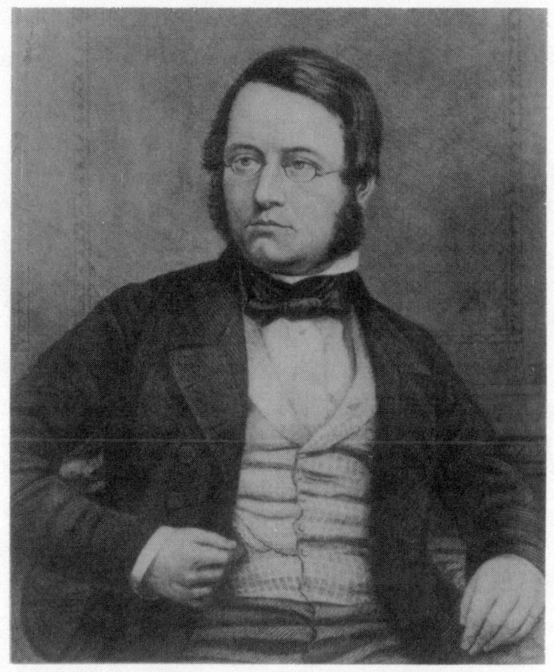

Sir Lyon Playfair   *(1818–1898)*

to get rid of women, that university even objected to being granted permissive powers to enable it to remedy the women's just grievances.

And so the battle raged. The newspapers joined too, and there were no holds barred. Sophia's "past" came back to haunt her as one newspaper noted that it was "amusing indeed that one of the ladies who had rendered herself most conspicuous should after all have failed under the test of examination." Edith Pechey wanted to rush to Sophia's defense, but she prudently held back.

Despite the efforts of Stansfeld and Cowper-Temple and others, the enabling bill was defeated, 196 to 153.

At the end of March, 1875, Cowper-Temple again took the initiative, but this time he tried a different approach. He introduced a bill entitled "Medical Acts Amendment (Foreign Universities) Bill." It called for recognition in Great Britain of medical degrees held by women graduates from universities in France and in Berlin, Leipzig, Bern, and Zurich. The medical faculties of universities of Britain opposed this bill on the ground that they could not be sure of the quality of the medical education carried on in the foreign universities. Taking its cue from the medical profession, the Government withheld its support too, and the bill was withdrawn in July.

There was, however, some progress. The feasibility, desirability, and advisability of admitting women to universities for medical education was a recurring theme in parliamentary debates through much of 1875. The Foreign Universities Bill focused attention on possible alternative solutions, although it posed a threat to the power and control of the General Medical Council over medical education. (This council, when asked for its opinion, had not come out bluntly against the women, but had piously warned that "the study and practice of medicine and surgery, instead of affording a field of exertion well fitted for women, do, on the contrary, present special difficulties which cannot be safely disregarded.") Moreover, the Government could no longer stand aside without leaving itself open to the serious charge of ignoring a social question that was assuming ever greater importance to the public.

As far as Queen Victoria was concerned, it was reported by the London *Times* that she laid the foundation stone for the new examination hall of the London College of Physicians and Surgeons in 1886. Did she know, did she care, did she even ask, one wonders, whether women were to be given the benefits of this college's medical training? (Women were not admitted to the college until 1909.) Perhaps it is significant that the year after the riot at Surgeons' Hall—1871—Queen Victoria conferred a baronetcy on Robert Christison. At worst she may have actually sided against the women in their fight to enter the medical profession, and at best perhaps she simply did not concern herself with such details; others in the Government would be left to deal with such matters.

At the end of July, 1875, Cowper-Temple questioned the Government spokesman about the official position on the whole matter and asked when legislation embodying that position would be presented to Parliament. The decision would be made known at the next session, was the reply. Cowper-Temple reminded the House that a medical school and a hospital were functioning in London in which doctors, teachers, and patients were women. But the women doctors were considered to be outlaws! Why? Because they held foreign degrees. And the British examining bodies, not recognizing these degrees, excluded the women from the examinations that would enable them to be licensed, included in the Medical Register, and thus given the legal right to practice medicine in Great Britain. The Medical Council now proposed new and special examinations for women, equal in quality to those for men.

The advocates of medical education for women had by 1876 developed a double plan of action. First, they tried to obtain recognition for degrees earned in foreign universities. Second, they attempted to get the nineteen examining boards to standardize their eligibility requirements as well as examinations.

Cowper-Temple took several opportunities to remind his listeners in the House of Commons that the 1858 Medical Reform Act used the word "persons" and did not exclude female as compared with male persons. In fact, two women had already been registered under this act—Elizabeth Blackwell and Elizabeth Garrett. The maneuver to exclude women must, therefore, he emphasized, be attributed to the examining bodies that changed their rules deliberately, as did the Apothecaries' Society. He reminded them, too, of the completely unethical behavior of the entire board of examiners in midwifery, and of the unwillingness of others to serve on a new board. All of this was contrived to thwart the spirit of the act of 1858 and to bar the way to women. England had closed its doors to them. Twelve of the twenty women then studying at the University of Paris were English, Scotch, or Irish. And so he was reintroducing the amendment he had previously proposed and withdrawn, which provided that holders of degrees from certain foreign universities could practice legally in Great Britain.

During the debate on this amendment support was forthcoming from another member, who cited some rather important statistics. According to the census of 1841 there were 15,800 practitioners in the population of 16,000,000. But in 1871 there were only 14,600 medical men in a population that had grown to 23,000,000 people. Moreover, the colonies around the globe had absorbed many physicians who might otherwise have remained at home. Parliament, by the harshness of law, placed women under many handicaps, which should be removed. Delaying the entrance of women into medical practice, the argument continued, was an injustice to the women who were studying and also to people who were suffering from various illnesses. Now was the time for action. It appeared that the Medical Council, the House, and the Government were at last in favor.

But the opponents were not yet ready to abandon the fight. Lower moral standards and lower educational standards were sure to be the result of women's admission to medicine, they argued. Even at that moment, the nineteen examining boards were lowering standards to attract candidates, because they depended largely on money received for giving their students a passing grade. Proper medical qualification required immediate attention, even before the question of admitting women could be considered. Cowper-Temple's bill contained ideas that were opposed to British notions of propriety. Furthermore, it was most unfortunate that "three or four ladies, by some means or other, had gotten their names into the Medical Register," but "hopefully, the number would never be increased!"

One of the early devices to delay action and stifle debate had been a motion to set up a Royal Commission on Scottish Universities to study the whole principle of public concern about women medical students. Lyon Playfair of the University of Edinburgh had proposed that motion, and he had been appointed to the commission. One of the conditions under which his motion was adopted was that responsible women would be given an opportunity to present their case. But the commission refused even to give the women a hearing. The four-volume report of that commission made only the most fleeting and casual reference—in the words of Dr. Robert Christison—to women candidates for medical degrees.

By 1876 the Government was primarily interested in seeing that the licensing bodies might be "allowed" to admit women to practice medicine and surgery, and in that case, perhaps Cowper-Temple would agree not to press for passage of the latest foreign universities amendment. Later in that session of Parliament an enabling bill entitled "Medical Act (Qualifications) Bill: to remove restrictions on granting of qualifications under the Medical Act on the grounds of sex and extend the power to grant qualification to all bodies under the Medical Act" was proposed with Government approval. The Medical Council added a condition, namely, that even if women were admitted to the Register, they would thereby not necessarily be qualified to take seats on the governing bodies of the university corporations. The bill was passed by Parliament, and finally, on August 11, 1876, royal assent was given. The historic bill was known as 39 and 40 Vict., c. 41.

Christison, still adamant, regarded the bill as almost a personal affront, viewing the wording of this "permissive" bill as a "newer device . . . to compel me to do that which my nature and reason detest, and which my *physique* declares it cannot sustain. . . . female practitioners are not wanted in this country. . . ."

Nonetheless, during the two years 1877 and 1878, Parliament tried to extend and improve the Medical Reform Act of 1858. Women's eligibility for medical education, but in classes separate from male students, was sanctioned. Their admission to examinations was to be followed by registration in the Medical Register. These conditions remained an essential part of all the legislation that was proposed. Many restrictions still remained. These were enforced to the extent that each individual examining body chose to use its option either to admit or not to admit women.

Several schemes were proposed in attempts to improve medical examinations and examining bodies, but the universities of Scotland rejected uncompromisingly and stubbornly all such proposals. To them, any and all legislation that favored women students of medicine or those in other fields as candidates for degrees was totally unacceptable.

The Medical Act of 1886, known as 49 and 50 Vict., c. 48, was the only one in the nineteenth century that came close to providing for uniform requirements for medical-degree candidates. But, even then, the admission of women to examinations still remained optional! Each particular examining body retained the right to make its own decision.

Parliament had indeed been of some service to our pioneering women medical students; it had made it clear that the word "persons" was meant to include women, and it had set the tone for a new and more enlightened attitude toward women in medicine. Progress would still be fairly slow, and, as ever, it would be largely up to the women themselves to look out for their own rights, even in the face of future parliamentary efforts to improve the medical profession.

Nonetheless, there were some heartening events to come. Thanks to the efforts of James Stansfeld, the University of London, after much debate, decided finally, in 1877, to admit women to its medical examinations; and early in 1878, it agreed to admit women to all degrees. The "hour of reform," as Stansfeld called it, seemed to be dawning.

According to Parliament, women could now be granted medical degrees, licensed, and included in the Medical Register. And in 1877 Edith Pechey and Sophia Jex-Blake became licensed physicians. What then happened to these leaders among the British women in medicine?

Now at last, with an M.D. and her name in the Medical Register, Sophia set her sights on the London School of Medicine for Women, which she had conceived, and to which she had virtually given life. She had up to now been only a trustee. Her degree was to be her key to the reward she had longed for so much, the position of Honorary Secretary, so that she might be officially recognized as such in the records of the school. She had done all the work connected with that office ever since the school had opened in October, 1874, but without any recognition. Then, as we have said, the objection of those she had admired for their achievements and reputations had prevented Sophia's name from being officially linked with the school's activities. But even now, there were still those who were convinced that it would be detrimental for the school to be closely associated with Sophia. So, she was taken at her words, uttered early in the school's life: "Put me utterly aside if need be!" Hard as it was for Sophia to see that "need" now, she stepped aside.

9.

The Final Outcome

Mrs. Thorne, one of the original five, and acceptable to everybody, had agreed to become Honorary Secretary, and although she had gotten an M.D., she put aside her own aspirations to practice medicine and made the success of the school her main object in life. In characteristic fashion, Sophia told her diary that Mrs. Thorne was "the best possible [choice], with her excellent sense and perfect temper. So much better than I!"

After some intensive soul-searching, and despite the need in London for women doctors, Sophia decided to start her professional career as a doctor—it's hard to believe—in Edinburgh, of all places! One would have thought that she would want to get as far away as possible from that city and some of the people who had caused her such heartache, anguish, and frustration for so many years. The riot at Surgeons' Hall had left such vivid memories in the mind of one of the women students that she said, some thirty years afterward, that on her occasional visits to Edinburgh, she would go miles out of her way rather than pass those gates of Surgeons' Hall. But not Sophia. Sophia had never really given up on Edinburgh. Finding the university unyielding, she had simply sought to realize her goal by taking a different path—which took her to London and Parliament, and to Ireland and Bern. And now that path led back to Edinburgh.

Already she had met with considerable success as a fledgling doctor. A patient in London had written to her: "What comfort it is to see your dear supporting face!" A patient to whom she had been called for an emergency visit quite early in her practice felt that when she came in "strong and swift, with your eagle's wings, getting over the distances in a third of the time other people take to do it," it was admirable treatment.

Sophia put up her shingle in June, 1878, at 4 Manor Street, the house she had taken when she decided to settle in Edinburgh. Her companions of earlier days—now qualified and practicing— had scattered far and wide. Edith Pechey was in Leeds. Isabel Thorne was in London at the school. How Sophia longed to have someone nearby with whom she could discuss difficult cases. She confided this to Mrs. Thorne in a letter written the following year: "I shall be really delighted if you will come down . . . and spend a week or two with me. . . . You and I have never had any really quiet time together since our student days, and I cannot tell you how much I should enjoy some talks with you, and how glad I should be for your advice about lots of things. . . . Dr. Sewall you know always said you were the doctor among us, and I quite believe it. I wish so very often that I could ask you about things." The doctors who had stood by Sophia in those difficult early years, now happily over, encouraged her to come to them whenever she felt the need, and—what was even more unusual in those days—they never ruled out any subject in medicine that they would have discussed with a man!

Sophia was a great success as a doctor in Edinburgh. Within three months after she settled there she started a small dispensary, and wrote her mother that "yesterday I received fees which just completed my first £50 [$250]—earned here in less than three months—and that in what they call the 'empty' season. And what pleases me still better is that every one of my patients has done well. Several have left my hands practically recovered, and those who are still there are all going on satisfactorily. And as among them were two cases to which I was called when the patient was described as 'dying' (and both got well), I think I may very well be content. I have had 23 patients (nearly 100 visits) at my private house, and about as many more in my Dispensary, which has only been open a fortnight; so I don't think there is much doubt about the 'demand' nor about my prospects."

In a letter to her old friend, Dr. King Chambers, she wrote: "I feel I am learning a great deal from the large variety of practice here. . . . I find that each of my cases involves so much reading and thinking that I am almost anxious they should not multiply too fast." Of course, there was much that Sophia was faced with in her practice that she wanted to learn about. Fortunately, as she also wrote Dr. King Chambers, "I have the help and support of four of the best medical men in Edinburgh, and they are all excessively kind in giving me advice and help as often as I want it."

To another doctor she wrote: "I have about 25 or 30 patients at the Dispensary every day that it is opened, and I also have a much larger private practice than is usual at so early a date. I have not yet been established here in practice quite 9 months, and I find that I have already had about 400 visits to or from private patients, which I think you will allow shows the 'demand' is a real one."

Evidently the doctor had raised some doubts in his letter to her about women in medicine. She was more than ready with her reply: "As you refer to the 'general question of lady doctors' you must allow me to say that I am quite sure it would have your support, from, at any rate, one point of view, if you had the least idea of the amount of preventable suffering which women bear with rather than consult men in special cases. . . . Now I do not care for a moment to argue whether this feeling is right or wrong; . . . if the feeling exists it should be distinctly recognized as an element in the question; and I am quite sure that you would be one of the very first to desire that every possible remedy should be brought to such needless suffering. In the same way I never care to argue at all about the relative capabilities of men and women. I mean to try to do my own work up to the very best of my power, and that is all that really concerns me. I cannot imagine any work nobler or more perfectly fascinating than that of medicine, and I am very thankful to be allowed ever so small a share in it."

If Sophia was finally winning the "Battle of Edinburgh," still not everyone had been won over to the idea of women in medicine. At about this time, when the University of London held a meeting to debate the admission of women students (which they agreed to do early in 1878), Sir William Jenner, one of the university's graduates, rose to give his opinion. He was an outstanding physician, had earlier won renown for distinguishing between typhus and typhoid fever, and was at that time "physician in ordinary" to Queen Victoria. A later historian of these events, E. Moberly Bell, described the scene this way: Jenner raised his hand to Heaven and "testified that he had but one dear daughter, and he would rather follow her bier to her grave than allow her to go through such a course of study" as medicine. (It seems that Victoria liked to surround herself with rather conservative physicians, for, as you may recall, another of her physicians was Sir Robert Christison.) As far as Sir William Jenner and his daughter were concerned, that young lady reacted naturally enough to the restraints of her upbringing and "did not sink into an early grave; on the contrary she became a robust and ardent suffragist. . . . " And, as a matter of fact, the young "she-doctors" who had grappled with Christison also became strong advocates of woman suffrage.

But the women's main efforts would have to remain on the medical front, for their victories were still fragile and easily endangered. For example, amendments to the latest medical bill were under consideration in Parliament in the fall of 1878. One sought to require that all doctors be qualified in both medicine and surgery. This was, no doubt, a move to upgrade medical education. But it concealed a threat to all the women who had already received their educations, for although the women had completed the surgical *training* required, since no college of surgeons would admit them to examinations, this change (which was later made the subject of a new bill) would in effect place those women doctors in an inferior position with respect to the men in the profession. Consequently, everything gained by the women up to that time would be lost to them. To add insult to injury, the General Medical Council proposed amendments to the new bill that would provide for a special board to give the women examinations and then place their names on a separate register! Furthermore, women would have to state that they had received *no part of their education with men.* This would immediately eliminate those women who were then studying at the University of Paris! Sophia realized that vigilance was still needed to safeguard what had been so dearly won. She wrote to Mrs. Garrett Anderson, asking her to urge those women doctors she knew to write a protest against the new bill and its amendments, to do so herself, and to try to get Dr. Elizabeth Blackwell to do likewise. Sophia sent along a draft of what she herself proposed for Mrs. Garrett Anderson's approval, comments, or improvements and urged that it be forwarded to James Stansfeld with a note that he alert others to the dangers in the new proposals. All of this was probably done, for some time later Sophia was able to tell Mrs. Thorne that she had heard from a Dr. Watson that "the Government is likely to drop the Medical Bill for this session." She also warned Mrs. Thorne to "make a point of 'keeping on the run' of every proposed amendment, and watching very carefully how each may affect women . . . [because] even friendly M.P.'s are too busy . . . and often they don't see the bearing of phrases" upon women's rights to practice.

Sophia and Edith Pechey and the rest of the little band were, fortunately, determined, resourceful women. Otherwise, who knows how much longer it might have been before their hopes were fulfilled? Both Sophia and Edith—and doubtless the others as well—had made for themselves extraordinary medical careers, fruitful and successful.

Sophia wrote a book, *Medical Women: A Thesis and a History,* which was published first in 1872 in—of course— Edinburgh. Later a revised version appeared in that city in 1886 as she was about to open her own hospital in Edinburgh for women and children, the very first of its kind in Scotland staffed by women and with women doctors at its head. Perhaps it is somewhat ironic that Dr. Christison's assistant, Mr. Craig, had a hand in this—for as we mentioned earlier, after the disastrous lawsuit, Sophia's supporters had actually raised a little more money than was needed to pay the court expenses. And Sophia had set aside the remainder for just this purpose—which she finally realized in 1886. She also founded a medical school for women in Edinburgh.

She searched for and finally found a suitable setting for her declining years. In November, 1898, she chose a ten-acre farm near the village of Mark Cross on the Forest Ridge of Sussex. She took possession the following May, began to raise all sorts of fruits and berries, and branched out into dairy farming, which she herself supervised. Her house was the meeting place (one visitor called it a mecca) for many of her former students and colleagues, for writers, and for friends from many parts of the world. Dr. Edith Pechey was among those most welcome at "Windydene," the name Sophia had chosen for her retreat.

When a recurring illness made surgery necessary, Sophia wanted two of her women students to operate but was dissuaded after she was told that it was unfair to place upon friends so great a responsibility. A compromise was worked out. Dr. Annie Clark, who had been a fellow student at Bern when Sophia and Edith Pechey received their medical degrees there in 1877, came from Birmingham to administer the anesthetic. Sophia was often prevented from sleeping by the pain caused by her illness, and she would say: "The worst of lying awake at night is that one realizes all the mistakes one has made in one's life." On January 9, 1912, she died; she was buried in the family grave site near Brighton, which, by a strange coincidence, is but a few yards from that of her old friend and champion, Sir James Stansfeld.

Edith Pechey found her major interest far from England and far from Edinburgh and Sophia. She went to India, arriving in Bombay in 1883. She had been invited by the Medical Women for India Fund to treat Indian women and girls, who were not allowed by religion and custom to be examined or treated by male doctors. At that time she was the very first fully qualified medical doctor who had no connection with religious missions. (Up until then, women missionaries had brought whatever incomplete medical knowledge they possessed to the women of India.) Edith Pechey's work in India was exceptionally significant, welcome to the poor who lived in the area where she opened her temporary dispensary, and rewarding. She married Herbert Phipson in India in 1889 and stayed there until 1905, when she retired and returned to England. She died three years later.

Matilda Chaplin, who had married her cousin, Professor William Edward Ayrton, had gone first to Paris, and then, when her husband was appointed to the Imperial College of Engineering in Tokyo, she went with him to Japan, where their daughter was born. They named her Edith—and we can wonder whether this was in honor, perhaps, of the brave Edith who had once been a classmate of Matilda Chaplin's. Mrs. Ayrton had continued her scientific work in Japan, and in 1879 she received her M.D. in Paris—ten years after she had first come to Edinburgh. She died shortly afterward, in 1883.

Isabel Thorne stayed on at the London School of Medicine for Women and wrote a history of it to 1904. Her daughter, May Thorne, became a doctor as well and carried on the family association with the London School.

Little is known of what happened to Helen (Evans) Russel, wife of *The Scotsman's* editor. She did apparently keep up her friendship with Sophia, for in 1885, the year before Sophia opened her Edinburgh hospital, Mrs. Russel paid her a visit. Sophia passed the news along to Edith Pechey that Mrs. Russel "was here for a few days a fortnight ago, and is as nice as ever."

If Edith had generally been considered more "acceptable" than the dauntless Sophia, still none of these women was really considered "womanly" in those days. Victorian tastes would have called for sweetness and charm, and put little premium on more aggressive qualities. These were girls who were driven by their own awareness of the needs of women for medical treatment and also for an opportunity to enter the medical profession. They were aware, too, of the intransigence of male physicians who, not dealing adequately with the medical needs of the female population, nonetheless sought to prevent women from becoming doctors in order to remedy this situation.

As Sophia put it, "mental equality" with men had not been the real issue: "I for one do not care in the least either to claim or disown such equality, nor do I see that it is at all essential to the real questions at issue. . . . We say to the authorities of the medical profession,—'. . . subject us ultimately to exactly the ordinary examinations and tests, and, if we fail to acquit ourselves as well as your average students, reject us; if, on the contrary, in spite of all difficulties, we reach your standard, and fulfil all your requirements, the question of "mental equality" is practically settled . . . leave the question of our ultimate success or failure in practice to be decided by ourselves and the public!'"

Perhaps if Sophia and Edith and the others had conformed more to Victorian models, the question of "mental equality" and the question of the women's ultimate success or failure would have been decided by Sir Robert Christison and Lyon Playfair.

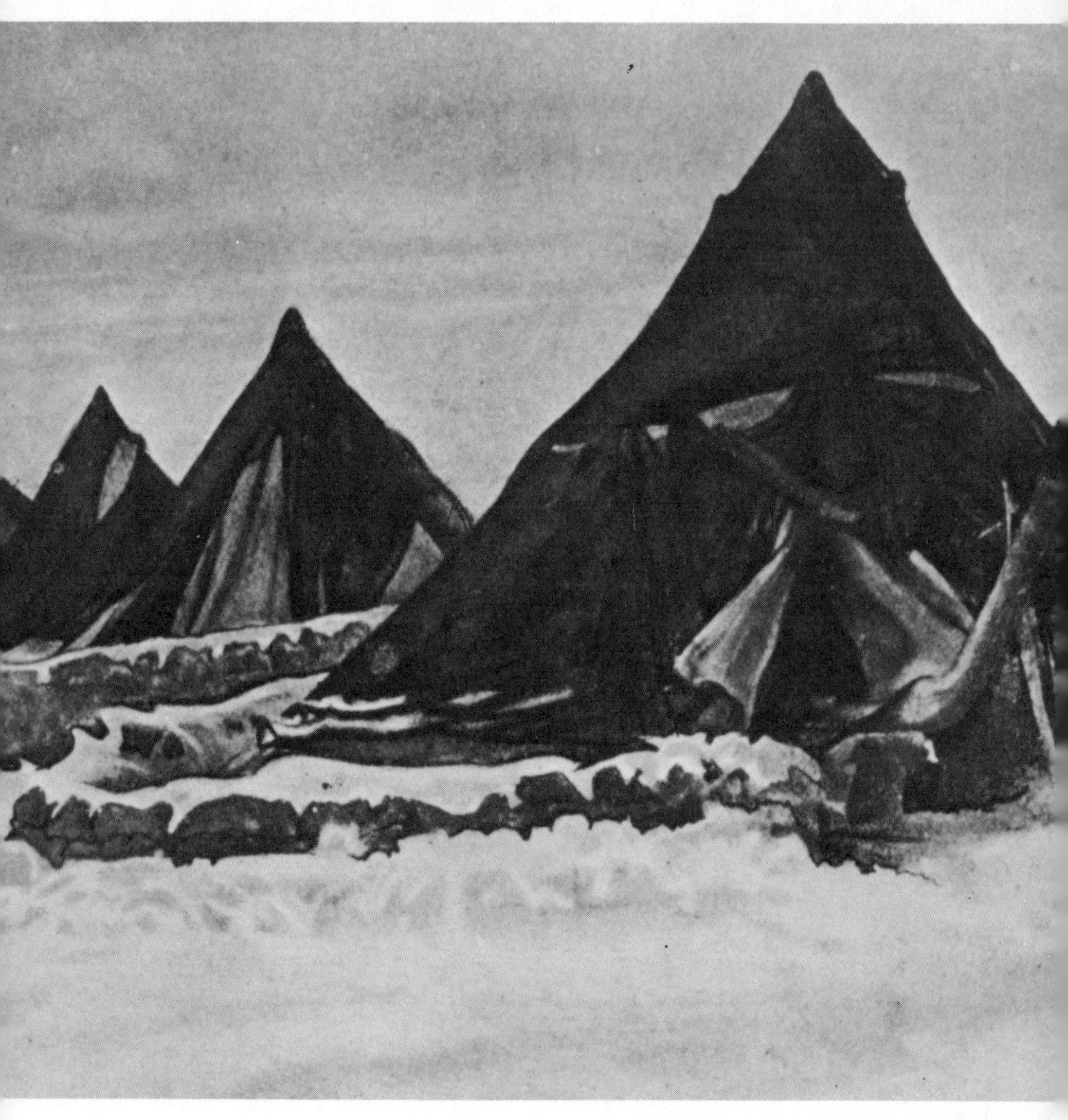

Military tents set up in the snow for clearing casualties during World War I

The period from 1869 to 1878 was a milestone in the advance of women in achieving the rights—professional, industrial, and political—that had been denied them from time immemorial. The immediate objective attained in this period was the right to study and practice medicine in Great Britain, a victory which had its repercussions throughout Europe and America.

In Britain, admitting women to the medical profession brought rather quick results. By 1881 there were twenty-five women doctors in England. And they continued to reflect the same high quality as the first women to seek a place in medicine. An undated report of the London School of Medicine for Women contains the statement that "at the Intermediate Examination in medicine of the University of London in August, 1881, Miss F. Helen Prideaux obtained the gold medal for anatomy, and Mrs. Scharlieb, Miss Tomlinson and Miss L. Bernard took honors in various other subjects."

At about this time one of the former Edinburgh students, Dr. Edith Shove, was appointed medical officer to the women post-office clerks. Sophia described this as "an immense step in public opinion."

In 1891 there were one hundred women doctors in England; twenty years later, more than two hundred; and in 1911, almost five hundred.

10.
Women in Medicine

The following year, 1912, Sophia Jex-Blake died. But she had seen her dream come true. The newspaper *The Queen* might have been speaking of her alone when it reported that "medical education of women has ultimately, owing to the strenuous exertions and steady perseverance of its advocates, been placed on an equality with men."

No doubt Sophia would have liked very much to hear the Vice Chancellor of the University of Edinburgh deliver the following remarks at the graduation ceremonies on October 23, 1926: "One very interesting item in the statistics that deserves more than passing mention," said the Vice Chancellor, "is the largely increased number of women in the University. Last year, out of 3,953 matriculated students, 1,911 were women. That is between one third and one quarter. In the Faculty of Arts, more than half of the number were women. In Science and Medicine the proportion was . . . much less, but there is no Faculty, not even Divinity . . . which escaped the invasion. . . . These figures are significant of a social change."

Some one hundred years ago a mere handful of women began their agitation at Edinburgh University. Since that time, and thanks in large part to that handful of women, others have entered the medical profession and often performed outstanding work. Dr. Annie McCall, who had been a student at the London School of Medicine for Women, started the first prenatal clinic for pregnant mothers in the 1880s. Another pioneer in maternity care was Dr. Janet Campbell, whose investigations and work in this field in the first quarter of the twentieth century contributed greatly to lowering the maternity death rate and the rate of infant mortality in Great Britain. She was honored with the title of D.B.E., Dame of the British Empire.

Dr. Jane Walker was a pioneer in the treatment of tuberculosis in Great Britain; Dr. Maude Abbott won renown for her work in heart disease. And during World War I, Dr. Elsie Inglis, a British doctor, went to Serbia (and then to other battlefronts as well), where, among other things, she organized tent hospitals as close to the fighting front as possible and became the heroine of untold numbers of wounded and sick soldiers. Dr. Hattie Alexander, a pediatrician in America, developed the first effective treatment of a form of meningitis that had previously been fatal for children. In 1964 she was president of the American Pediatric Society, one of the few women ever to head a major medical society. And Dr. Janet Travell gained national prominence as personal physician to President John F. Kennedy.

Hardly an exhaustive list, these are just a few of the many names of outstanding women doctors. And perhaps, too, we should mention Dorothy Hodgkin, of Great Britain, who won the Nobel Prize in Chemistry in 1964. A change indeed from Edith Pechey's troubles over a less renowned chemistry prize in 1870.

There have been many changes. In the United States, for example, the number of women in medical work of all kinds was 7,400 in 1900. Thirty years later, in 1930, the number had risen to 20,000. In Great Britain, according to recent figures, the women who were full-time students of pure and applied science, medicine, and also of dentistry, agriculture and forestry, veterinary science, and social studies, numbered almost 18,000.

Perhaps it is an irony of history that if you wanted to visit the London School of Medicine for Women today, you wouldn't find it. In 1944, when England was considering the formation of a national health service, a committee was appointed to investigate medical schools. The report of this committee, known as the Goodenough Report, after the name of the committee's chairman, recommended that Government grants to any medical school be given only if certain conditions were met, one of them being that the school must be coeducational. And so it was that the London School of Medicine for Women opened its doors—to men! And the name of the school was changed to the Royal Free Hospital School of Medicine.

If the admission of women to medical schools is not the problem today that it was for Sophia and her band, still the number of women medical students in relation to male students is small. Today only 7 percent of the physicians in America are women, although the percentage is far higher in many other countries. Raising that percentage—here and elsewhere—is one of the many challenges still to be met.

It will be today's young women who will forge tomorrow's paths for women in medicine.

Suggested Further Reading

Anderson, Louisa Garrett. *Elizabeth Garrett Anderson: 1836–1917*. London, 1939.

Aveling, James Hobson. *The Chamberlens and the Midwifery Forceps*. London, 1882.

Bell, Enid Hestor Chataway Moberly. *Storming the Citadel: The Rise of the Woman Doctor*. London, 1953.

Blackwell, Elizabeth. *Pioneer Work in Opening the Medical Profession to Women*. London, 1895.

Jex-Blake, Sophia. *Medical Women: A Thesis and a History*. Edinburgh, 1872. 2nd ed. revised, Edinburgh, 1886.

Kerr, John Munro, and others. *Historical Review of British Obstetrics and Gynaecology: 1800–1950*. Edinburgh, 1954.

Lovejoy, Dr. Esther Pohl. *Women Doctors of the World*. New York, 1957.

Mead, Kate Campbell-Hurd. *A History of Women in Medicine*. Conn., 1938.

Murray, Dr. Flora. "The Position of Women in Medicine and Surgery." *New Statesman*, London, Vol. II (1913–1914), Nov. 1, 1913, Special Supplement, pp. xvi-xvii.

Phipson, Edith Pechey. *Address to the Hindoos of Bombay on the Subject of Child Marriage*. Delivered at the Hall of the Prarthana Somaj, Bombay, on 11 October, 1890, Butler Library, Columbia University.

Russel, M. P. "James (Miranda?) Barry." *Edinburgh Medical Journal*, Vol. I (1943), pp. 558–567.

Rutherford, Col. N. J. C. "James (Miranda?) Barry." *Journal of the Royal Army Medical Corps*. London, Vol. XCVI–XCVII (May, 1951), pp. 278–281.

Stansfeld, James. "Medical Women," *Nineteenth Century*, London, Vol. I, No. 5 (July, 1877), pp. 888–901.

Stoddart, Anna M. *Elizabeth Pease Nichol.* London, 1899.

Strachey, Ray. *The Cause: A Short History of the Women's Movement in Great Britain.* London, 1928.

Thorne, Mrs. Isabel. *Sketch of the London School of Medicine for Women.* London, 1905.

Todd, Margaret. *The Life of Sophia Jex-Blake.* London, 1918.

Young, G. M. *Victorian England: Portrait of an Age.* London, 1936.

ACKNOWLEDGMENTS

This book has been the result of extensive research, especially into the history of medical education for women in Great Britain. Whenever it was necessary to consult primary sources, as in the case of parliamentary debates, reports of royal commissions, minutes of the Irish College of Physicians, enrollment records of the University of Bern in Switzerland, to mention a few, I have done so.

I wish to thank the following libraries, journals, and authors for their valuable help in preparing this work and for permission, whenever it was required, to quote or reproduce illustrations: *Association Medical Journal,* London; Enid Moberly Bell, *Storming the Citadel,* London, 1953; *Bicentenary of the Faculty of Medicine, 1726-1926,* University of Edinburgh, Edinburgh, 1926; *British Medical Journal;* The British Museum, London; Columbia University Libraries, New York City; Edinburgh University Library and Manuscript Division; *Encyclopaedia Britannica,* 11th edition; Fawcett Library, London; General Medical Council, London; Dr. Douglas Guthrie of Edinburgh; Irish College of Physicians, Dublin; Sophia Jex-Blake, *Medical Women: A Thesis and a History,* Edinburgh, rev. ed., 1866; John Munro Kerr and others, *Historical Review of British Obstetrics and Gynaecology: 1800-1950,* Edinburgh, 1954; *The Lancet,* London; *Life and Letters* (autobiography of Thomas Henry Huxley) edited by his son, Edinburgh or London; *Life of Robert Christison,* by his son, Edinburgh or London; *The London Illustrated News,* London; London School of Medicine for Women, London, now Royal Free Hospital School of Medicine; the late Dr. Douglas McKie, London; The New York Academy of Medicine; *The Scotsman,* Edinburgh; Dr. Richard H. Shryock, American Philosophical Society, Philadelphia, Pennsylvania; Sophia Smith Collection, Smith College: Director, Margaret S. Grierson; Margaret Todd, *The Life of Sophia Jex-Blake,* London, 1918; The University of Bern Library; The Wellcome Historical Medical Library, London; Women's Archives, Radcliffe College, Cambridge.

Partial help was given by the American Philosophical Society of Philadelphia, Pennsylvania, to whom I am especially grateful for the confidence they expressed in awarding me the first grant of funds I ever received, in 1965.

Special appreciation is due to Dr. Daniel Greenberg, whose constant and continuous encouragement sustained me during several periods of near-despair. This effort was enhanced by the cooperation and understanding extended by my husband, Philip, when the going was difficult, and by my three sons, three daughters-in-law, and grandsons, who refrained from making demands upon me so that I could continue with a clear conscience.

Accuracy and the search for truth have been my aims. If I have fallen short of these, I bear that responsibility alone.